Dragonfly

Dragonfly

A DAUGHTER'S EMERGENCE FROM AUTISM
A Practical Guide for Parents

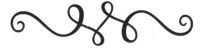

LORI ASHLEY TAYLOR
FOREWORD BY JENNIFER O'TOOLE

Skyhorse Publishing

Skyhorse Publishing books may be purchased in bulk at special discounts for sales promotion, corporate gifts, fund-raising, or educational purposes. Special editions can also be created to specifications. For details, contact the Special Sales Department, Skyhorse Publishing, 307 West 36th Street, 11th Floor,
New York, NY 10018 or info@skyhorsepublishing.com.

Skyhorse® and Skyhorse Publishing® are registered trademarks of Skyhorse Publishing, Inc.®, a Delaware corporation.

Visit our website at www.skyhorsepublishing.com.

10 9 8 7 6 5 4 3 2 1

Library of Congress Cataloging-in-Publication Data is available on file.

Cover design by Rain Saukas
Cover photo © 2015 by Andrea Moberly

ISBN: 978-1-5107-3217-9
Ebook ISBN: 978-1-5107-3218-6

Printed in the United States of America

To Hannah and Connor
I would move mountains for the both of you.

To All Special Needs Families
Hope is the catalyst for our children to live their best lives. Without hope, there is only fear.

I suspect the truth is that we are waiting, all of us, against insurmountable odds, for something extraordinary to happen to us.
—Khaled Hosseini

contents

Author's Notes   xi

Foreword   xiii

Prologue   xvii

Introduction   xix

Meet the Ladies of Wisdom from the Round Table   xxv

Timeline   xxix

Chapter One: The "D" Word (Diagnosis/Identification)   1

Chapter Two: Life before Autism   15

Chapter Three: Something's Not Quite Right (Early Signs
    and Worries)   25

Chapter Four: Rewriting the Script (The Earliest Interventions)   39

Chapter Five: A Baby Boy is Born (Sibling Relationships)   63

Chapter Six: Strength in Numbers (The Power of
    Community)   83

Chapter Seven: Changing Normal (Stage Two Interventions)   101

Chapter Eight: Holidays and Vacations   129

Chapter Nine: Flying Solo (Single Motherhood)   149

Chapter Ten: Both Sides of the Table
    (Meeting Students' Educational Needs)   169

Chapter Eleven: Find Your Warriors   189

Chapter Twelve: Autism Anecdotes   203

Chapter Thirteen: Acceptance and Fostering Independence   223

Chapter Fourteen: A New Day   253

Epilogue   269

Appendix: Glossary, Endnotes, Suggested Resources,
   and Index   271

Acknowledgments   293

About the Author   295

author's notes

All bolded words have been defined in the glossary.

Some names and identifiable details have been changed to protect people's privacy.

Dragonfly was written to address both genders of children with autism, so pronouns will alternate.

Dragonfly uses the "identity first" phrasing when describing individuals with a disability. Thus, "a boy with autism" is used rather than "an autistic boy." Some groups and advocates such as those in the neurodiversity movement prefer the latter. I mean no disrespect and hope this doesn't create a barrier to any readers—in fact, I hope we can overcome our differences and instead join forces to learn from one another.

Functioning level language (high-functioning or low-functioning) has only been used where the content requires specific language to be accurately understood. According to diagnostic criteria, high-functioning relates to Level 1, **Diagnostic and Statistical Manual of Mental Disorders, Fifth Edition (DSM-5) criteria**, and low-functioning relates to Level 3, DSM-5 criteria. By no means am I suggesting an individual's functioning or potential should be limited—as you may have noted from the book's title and what you'll see as soon as you read the first few chapters. I encourage parents to think in terms of emergence rather than limits—my goal is to help as many parents as possible with kids at every level of the autism spectrum, and it's difficult to talk about a

specific level on the spectrum without having a shorthand terminology.
I also understand that this simple dichotomy is not exact, as development is multidimensional and individuals are uniquely complex. My
intention is to avoid offending—if at all possible. I only use this terminology to try to open the conversation, so instead of shutting down the
conversation in disagreement over terminology, let's join in a place of
common ground with a shared goal of seeing each child reach his full
potential.

Likewise, the term "emergence" used in the subtitle and throughout
the text refers to meeting and overcoming some of the challenges that
make it difficult to function within our world. A shared, universal conviction of parents is that we all want the absolute best quality of life for
our children, which includes helping individuals with autism become
as independent as possible. The connotation shouldn't be inferred that
autism is a dreadful, lurid place that one needs to escape. *Dragonfly* is
not about a cure or fix from autism, nor is about recovery from autism.
It is simply about embracing autism and helping to build the best life
possible for our children.

foreword

Being the new kid on the block is tough. Disorienting. Sometimes lonely. You can't remember the unfamiliar words in the address, you don't know anybody, and you may be more than a little overwhelmed by all of the advice you get from neighbors, both old and new. And everyone seems to have an opinion about the place. It's ok. We get it. We know this may not be where you expected to find yourself and that unfamiliar can be scary.

On the other hand, new surroundings can mean fresh beginnings. A new school, university, job, house, relationship—each offers a way to totally reinvent yourself. In the process, you may well have discovered "your people." The crowd who just seemed to "get" you without loading you up with a "rep" full of expectations and limitations. You got to be you...only you-i-er.

Welcome, friend. Here, we *are* different. We are different—together.

Autism isn't for sissies. As a seven-time author, international speaker, former teacher, counselor, a mother of three children on the spectrum, and someone who was, myself, diagnosed only seven years ago, I know, first-hand, that "different" is tough stuff for everyone involved. In so many ways, each of us feels unseen. Unheard. We feel desperate to know we are doing the right thing. And guilty for wishing, sometimes, that life had dealt us an easier hand. In just the last five years, I've had the privilege of keynoting before tens of thousands of people the world over. All of us share intersecting journeys. Yet all of us, at one point or another, believe that we are completely and utterly alone.

We aren't. You aren't. Around here, you are the perfectly imperfect norm. Not alone in a crowd. Recognized and welcomed by it.

This past summer, my daughter and I were in Wisconsin, at the Autism Society of America's national conference. Late one afternoon, just after John Elder Robison, Stephen Shore, Alex Plank and I had finished a photo op with the attendees, I overheard a woman bubble to her friend, "Those are all the famous people!" How odd, I thought. An autism self-advocate version of the Justice League. To many people, I suppose that sort of ego boost would feel like an arrival of sorts. A triumph. An emergence. To me, though, that afternoon wasn't about being known to a crowd. It was about being known to one little girl. Hannah.

From across the conference center lobby, I heard a high-pitched squeal and turned to see a young girl bouncing excitedly on her toes. Her hands were clenched with a sense of thrill, her smile brimming from ear to ear. Beside her, a woman, presumably her mother, was equally giddy. "That's her, Hannah! That's Jennifer! Go ahead—go over!"

Moments later, I was stunned to discover that all of the fuss was over me. That one of my books, *Sisterhood of the Spectrum,* was her absolute favorite. That I was her "heroine." Which was ridiculous, I explained . . . because *she wa*s the heroine. The star of her own life story. And now, I got to be *her* fan.

Lori Taylor tells me that we first met several years ago at a talk I'd given in Colorado. The truth is, though, that I don't remember the occasion. It's not that she is forgettable—not in the least. It's just that the people who star in my memory are the children. Over the course of the conference, Lori and I *did* get to know one another well. So, recently, when Lori asked me to contribute the foreword, I was honored.

Honored to be here for my Maura, Sean, and Gavin. For Hannah. And for the heroes in *your* life story.

Dragonfly is the kind of "keeping it real" story I believe in because Lori knows that "emerging from autism," isn't about escaping a life sentence or overcoming a tragedy. It's triumphing stigma. And ignorance. And judgement. And grief. It's stepping out of the distorted image the world has of autism, and stepping into the sun. Into the un-expected wonderful that autism can be. She and her work in this book are the embodiment of what I call "relentless positivity." The kind that chooses to keep going. To be afraid and do it anyway. To inspire by vul-nerability as much as credibility.

I've heard it said that we should walk gently through this world, remembering that each one is fighting her own battle. I'd like to think that instead of fighting, we are each thriving. Striving. Dreaming. Only when others are hard, presumptuous, or judgmental must we fight ceaselessly for peace and dignity. In the pages ahead, you will read personal stories that will leave you thinking, "That's terrible! *I'd* never do *that*!" Yet every one of us "does that." When we haven't patience, humility or presence-of-mind, our best selves, it seems, become invis-ible, too.

I know "right now" may be hard. I know it from the bottom of my soul. So does Lori. So does Hannah. I also know—as someone whose world has only ever been an autistic world—that each of our children is a wonderful occasion. More than a one-in-a-million kind of kid. They are each a once-in-a-lifetime kind of person. And we get to love them.

As you read, look for ways in which you might love more abun-dantly, live more generously. Be kinder to yourself. See us as being, first, on the human spectrum. Listen. Don't argue back, even in thought. Just listen. And above all, have a bit more faith in one another. Faith is, after all, the belief in things unseen...in invisible beauty. Read on. Wonder if there's more than meets the eye. Because there is. There always is. And you can only see it with your heart.

There is a parable, whose author is unknown, which perfectly sum-marizes my view of the world. It tells of a woman who awakes to find only three hairs on her head. She smiles and says, "I think I'll braid my hair today." The next day, she discovers only two hairs, and gladly proclaims that today, she will part her hair down the middle! On the third morning, she spies one hair left, and laughs, "I will wear a pony-tail today!" And when at last she wakes to find no hairs remaining, she joyfully announces, "Yay! I don't have to do my hair today!"

Life begins at the edge of our comfort zones, I have heard. And if that's the case, that is the whole world for us, living on the spectrum. Which I'd say means that we'd better stick together. There's a whole lot of living to do.

PROLOGUE

why dragonfly?

"Mommy! Mommy! Look what I made!"

I place one of the last moving boxes on the kitchen floor and sit at the table. I'm worn out having to do this all by myself. As I glance at the clock on the stove, I see that two hours have elapsed since I began. Hannah has kept herself busy writing and drawing for some time. She's finally used one of the blank booklets I made for her to write a story. A yellow-and-pink (her favorite colors) dragonfly with silver wings and bulging eyes graces its cover. She places a solitary piece of lined paper in front of me. The writing appears to be in stanza form and continues onto the back. Apparently, the blunt pencil scratching the paper didn't bother her.

It was June 2013, and Hannah, my eight-year-old with autism, had beckoned me into her world—a rare and precious occasion. Each time it happens, Hannah's extraordinary perspective is revealed and I'm privileged to view the world through her lens. My daughter gleans meaning and makes associations that others would not consider or propose.

On that day Hannah handed me two literary works of art that I will treasure more than the classics that have adorned my bookshelves over the ages. The first piece was an illustrated short story entitled "The Lost Dragonfly." The second piece was a poem in free verse called "Life as a Dragonfly." The elements of theme and metaphor reflected in her short story were amplified further in her poem by the use of structure, parallelism, rhythm, and repetition. Hannah's profound sense of self-awareness astonished me. Clearly, one does not need to be a wordsmith to identify this behavior as a different ability versus a disability.

Hannah, like so many others with autism, has an innate and sacred connection with nature. However, it was still a surprise that this brightly colored insect would inspire my anxious yet precocious little girl to liken its arduous, transformative journey to hers.

Many people are unfamiliar with the maturation cycle of the common dragonfly. Being a science teacher and a Department of Natural Resources volunteer, I knew all about how female dragonflies will release their eggs into ponds or marshy areas because the waters are calm. The eggs then hatch to reveal the unrecognizable nymphs. The dragonfly may actually spend two to four years in the water before emerging to take flight.

In "The Lost Dragonfly," Hannah had already made her way into our world—that is, the dragonfly that represented her had emerged above water. However, the creature did not possess **social pragmatics** and felt alone. Her dragonfly tried to befriend fireflies, moths, and worms without any luck. In "Life as a Dragonfly," Hannah used paralleled and repeated stanzas that mirrored her physical and cognitive development with the dragonfly's actual stages of life. The most poignant words: "Hope rises, and I begin to reveal my concealed wings. I begin to understand language and what I am meant to do."

Before long, the dragonfly became more than a symbol for change and renewal—for us, it grew to become a regal symbol for Hannah's courage to break the water's surface and fly after so much time. She emerged even though the wind at times was and can still be tumultuous. Dragonflies have now seemed to appear in our darkest of hours. Their appearance has provided solace in times when our spirits could have easily withdrawn. It's easy to see why they are considered the keepers of dreams, the energy within that sees all of our true potential and ability. They remind us that anything is possible.

introduction

When the world says "give up," hope whispers, try one last time.
—KERRY MAGRO

May 2006
I wave goodbye to my thirty-two sixth graders, pick up my daughter,
Hannah, and we begin our forty-five-minute commute home. Hannah
is squirming in her car seat and wailing so hard she sounds like she's
gagging. My knuckles are white on the wheel.

"Keep it together," I tell myself. "Keep it together for everyone. For
Hannah."

Isn't that what working moms are supposed to do?

Our daycare provider told me Hannah wouldn't eat again today.
And then she said Hannah's lost her ability to pull up ever since she
had that upper respiratory infection, croup, and bilateral ear infections
in early spring. Our doctor had treated her with antibiotics and ster-
oids. I try to loosen my grip on the wheel. I take a deep breath to relax.
That's what my friend said I should do to relax, as if one breath could
make a difference.

By the time I pull into the garage, I realize Hannah has quieted
down. I wipe the smeary mess of tears off Hannah's face, then lift her
out of the car seat to get inside. I glance at the kitchen clock—my

husband will be home within the hour. I should get some sort of din-
ner started.

I position Hannah in front of her toy box and flip on the television.
As I start to walk away, I hear the anchorman from CNN Headline
News: "Imagine your child has just received a diagnosis of autism . . .
that would be a tragedy for any family."

A tragedy?

Am I living a tragedy? My daughter's not eating and can't pull her-
self up and shrieks all the way home. And that's just today's challenges.
Is that a tragedy? I don't know, but I'm hit hard.

I can't . . . I can't hear anything else the man says. My heart pounds,
and I drop to the couch a few feet away from the television and Han-
nah. I pull my knees in close and lie on my side. As I bring my hand to
my mouth, long-suppressed emotions release. Tears start to soak my
skirt, and I can't stop, and my face is as smeared with tears as Hannah's
was in the car.

After who knows how long, the sobbing slows, and I'm aware that
Hannah still sits in the same spot but has not witnessed my agony. She
is simply "not there."

Is this tragic? I lost the daughter I thought I had. She's different.
Our family is different. Her life is going to be hard, so hard . . . so, so
hard. And I can't stop crying.

Over ten years ago my family was hit with the life-altering diagnosis of
autism. I say *family* because when a member of the family is diagnosed
with autism, it affects the entire unit. Autism had confined my oldest
child, Hannah, to an inaccessible world. Blindsided by the news, we
struggled to see a bright side.

At the age of eighteen months, Hannah was diagnosed with
low-functioning autism. Though I never cared for the term "low-
functioning," I can see why the medical community began using it in
relation to the kinds of symptoms they saw in Hannah: no babbling or
talking, no walking, periodic **stimming** (self-stimulating behavior), lack
of eye contact, sensitivity to touch and sound, a **failure to thrive**, and

more. Her neurologist's prognosis gave a slim chance of her ever being mainstreamed into a general education classroom.

Autism is a mysterious developmental disorder affecting more than three and a half million Americans. It's the world's fastest growing developmental disability. There is no proven cause or cure, and families living with autism will attest to the devastation caused by this disorder. The word *autism* is a Greek derivative of *autos*, meaning extremely self-aware. Individuals with autism often appear to be self-absorbed—making it difficult for them to interact with the outside world. The hallmark symptoms of autism include challenges in social communication (both verbal and nonverbal), challenges in social interaction (the ability to cultivate and maintain friendships), and restricted, repetitive patterns of behavior, interests, or activities (such as sensory challenges, fixated and intense interests, a "need" for strict routines, and repetitive or odd motor movements). Autism occurs in all ethnic and socioeconomic groups. When we were told Hannah's diagnosis, I had been teaching for fourteen years and was pregnant with our second child, Connor. The minute the doctor uttered the word autism, I felt our dreams slipping away—dreams of a healthy child who would grow up to marry and enjoy a gratifying career and have babies of her own. For Hannah, that all seemed impossible. The doctor told me she might need my help to do the simplest tasks all the way into her adulthood.

But I held onto something. Maybe it was foolish of me. Maybe it was prescience. Maybe it was exactly what she and I needed most of all.

Hope.

Hope helped me keep it together. I had hope that she'd catch up—that she would prove those doctors wrong. Hope helped me reject any other alternative. Hope for her progress stretched my perspective and changed me. I've heard people say you can let a pivotal, adverse moment define, destroy, or strengthen you. Our pivotal moment strengthened me. In fact, our entire journey has brought more and more strength both to me and to Hannah.

After Hannah's identification, I read anything and everything I could get my hands on to educate myself as fast as possible. Before her diagnosis, I had no idea autism was on the rise, that the Centers for Disease Control had ruled autism an epidemic in the United States.

Over my years as a teacher, only a few of my students were on the autism spectrum, and they were all high-functioning—again, I dislike the terminology, as there may be more effective ways to identify people, and in my case specifically students, who are able to integrate effectively into social settings and do the required work alongside typical students. I only knew a few families who had children with more severe challenges. The information I gleaned from those books shaped me into a staunch advocate for my daughter. I learned about the plasticity of the brain and the need to provide early intervention during a narrow window of time. We were in a race against time, but never underestimate the power of a parent fighting to save her child.

I spearheaded an entourage of therapists and doctors to try everything possible to help Hannah. After five years of courage, persistence, hard work, and dedication, our continuous intervention did pay off. In some cases, a child can progress and shift on the autism spectrum, and Hannah has done just that.

I forged my way into my daughter's world, pulled her into my world, and loved her back to herself. It's important to note that I didn't ask Hannah to come into my world without first visiting hers. "Off in her own world" was certainly not cliché for daydreaming. Children with autism seem to ignore us, but that's simply not the case. They're waiting for us to enter their world. Over time I learned to focus on Hannah's strengths and passions, but I also didn't deny either of us traditional play. Contemporary American author Diane Ackerman said, "Play is our brain's favorite way of learning." Among other effective techniques and approaches, you'll see the role of occupational therapy in minimizing Hannah's **sensory processing disorder**, which most often goes hand in hand with autism. We gently stepped in and met Hannah in the way she thinks and feels and processes the world.

Just as some dragonflies take years and years to emerge, so did my daughter. Every single child needs a champion to see him through that process. I became Hannah's champion. We saw her emerge, but that doesn't mean Hannah no longer has autism. The miracle cure I desperately longed for did not appear. There is no cure. Hannah will always have the attributes that defined her autism in the first place;

however, her level of functioning with all of those behaviors has greatly improved.

At the time of this writing, Hannah is twelve years old and is in our school system's High Ability Program. In the current DSM-5, she would be identified as having autism only, but she was labeled as having a form of autism formerly known as **Asperger's syndrome**, which many in the autism community continue to use as an effective description. Hannah still faces some huge social and emotional challenges, but with her resiliency and drive I know she will accomplish great things.

I pray that the most important suggestions in this book resonate with every reader: have hope, lose the pride and denial, implement early intervention, and don't allow grief to zap your energy.

Over the years, I would read outstanding memoirs written by champion parents with special needs children, but struggled to find the commonalities between those children and Hannah. Yes, the ones with autism shared the same diagnosis criteria, but if you have a loved one with autism, this will ring true: "You know one child with autism, you still only know one child with autism." In other words, it's almost impossible to gather universally applicable truths or realities for families dealing with an autism diagnosis, but in *Dragonfly*, I intend to try. I want to offer readers not only stories but also useful resources valuable to every parent.

As a teacher, I know how powerful resources can be and have seen students in my classroom who have **Individual Education Plans** (IEPs) flourish simply because their needs are being met with all they need to succeed. I'm not providing you with an individualized plan, but I do intend to give you inspiration and ideas to succeed. As a teacher, I understand what it's like to work with students who are struggling with special needs, including autism; as a parent, I understand your side of the table. I'm in the trenches with you.

Here's how to get the most out of this book.

First, each chapter contains text boxes that offer strategies for a wide range of challenges that parents with a child on the spectrum must face—and perhaps overcome. These text boxes are available as a quick reference guide.

Next, even though readers may connect with something in Hannah's experiences, I offer them a variety of examples in hopes they can find traits that mirror those of their own child. To achieve that goal, I sat down with six mothers who have children of all ages and ranges on the autism spectrum. I asked them six integral questions that any parent with a child on the spectrum would long to hear the answers to. If you met others facing similar challenges, you'd probably ask these questions yourself. Take time to read through their wise, loving responses shared at the end of each chapter in a section called "Wisdom from the Round Table." Meet the moms and see the questions I posed to them on the next page.

In the appendix, you'll find a glossary. When I first started helping Hannah, I needed a glossary of terms on hand any time I attended a doctor's appointment, workshop, or convention, because professionals tossed out jargon I had never encountered. What is **theory of mind** and why does Hannah have such a difficult time determining what another person is thinking or feeling? Who ever heard of **executive functioning** and why can't Hannah follow a verbal list or stay organized? I've captured and defined many key terms you'll encounter, to accelerate your understanding so you can more quickly engage with the professionals involved in your child's treatments. You might even want to add them to a note on your phone so your personal autism lexicon can grow over time and always be on hand.

By sharing our personal journey, I hope you'll find hope in the story, answers in the content, and comfort in the prose. I feel my experience, knowledge, and understanding will benefit your own journey. Personally, I feel a driven mother's passion to encourage tangible actions that yield positive results. Let me be a voice to strengthen you on the hard days. Don't give up. There is no false hope. Sometimes a parent needs to know that whatever seems impossible can become a reality.

By the way, the word "dragonfly" in certain cultures means joy is in the journey. Inspirational writer and lecturer Joseph Campbell said, "Find the place inside where there is joy, and the joy will burn out the pain."

You will find joy again. Let's journey together.

meet the ladies
of wisdom from the round table

Six experienced and respected mothers gathered at a local restaurant in a private, candlelit room one evening to share their insight, experience, and staunch advocacy for their children with autism in order to help others that follow. Their children ranged in age from thirteen to twenty-three, and each child represented a different level of the autism spectrum.

Most of the mothers had been navigating the journey for years—some of them for decades. These women shared a bond understood best by others with similar struggles, which is why I chose them as spokespersons. As they answered the questions I posed, stories and advice poured out that prompted celebration of accomplishments and tears of frustration.

The six thought-provoking questions below provided the focus for the evening, and as they revealed truths surrounding autism, I documented their answers to share them with you. At the close of each chapter, you'll read excerpts from our conversation as we welcome you to the virtual round table. You'll soon see that you're not alone.

Let's meet Lori R., Jen, Lori V., Susan, Karen, Sarah, and their families.

Lori R. will be sharing her family's journey with their sunshine boy, Cameron (nineteen), who lights up a room when he walks in. Diagnosed with autism at the age of three, Cameron has just completed high school. He has an older brother in graduate school, a sister in college, and a seventeen-year-old brother. Lori and her husband, Steve, just completed the process of obtaining legal guardianship for Cameron, because he is not capable of making his own medical and financial decisions. Lori believes that God has used Cameron to strengthen their family's faith and to teach them life lessons. She knows they are a better and a closer family because of Cameron. Cameron enjoys a hard workout at the YMCA and can often be found on the treadmill or stair climber.

Jen will encourage your spirit with her contagious, positive, and matter-of-fact outlook on raising her son, Noah (nineteen), who was diagnosed with autism at the age of two. Noah works for McAlister's Deli, where he is known as the cookie guy. Jen and her husband, Ryan, view their situation with the belief that God had different plans for Noah, which meant different plans for them, too. From the point of diagnosis on, Jen has always been Noah's champion advocate. As he transitions to adulthood, Jen looks forward to seeing which doors open for Noah, trusting God's guidance.

Lori V. not only tirelessly advocates for her son, Byron (twenty-two), who has Asperger's syndrome, but she helps others become aware of their child's educational opportunities and rights. Byron was diagnosed with autism the summer after second grade. He has always been interested in the sciences and has always acted as a "little professor." Byron has been mainstreamed into the High Ability Program his entire school career. He has a younger brother, Devin (twenty), who is a junior in college. Lori quit her job when Byron was diagnosed with autism and then several years later went through a painful divorce. Byron has always gotten stuck in the cracks because he has trouble fitting in and making friends, and they found it was too challenging for Byron to be away at college by himself, so he's going to try to continue his education part-time while living at home.

Susan and her husband, Bruce, knew their son Tyler (twenty-three) had difficulties when he was just six months old. Tyler's initial diagnosis was developmental delay, then developmental delay with cerebral palsy, then autism with moderate cognitive disability and cerebral palsy. Susan was a special education teacher and is now a school psychologist. Tyler, who is nonverbal, was in a Life Skills Program throughout his school career and, most recently, moved into a waiver home. Even though Tyler can be a very loving and sweet boy, Susan's family struggled with managing his behaviors. Susan's daughter, Allie (twenty-five), has been through many emotions with her brother. Allie loves him and will be his legal guardian when the time comes. Through her professional and parental roles, Susan attempts to help all families from preschool through adulthood make the best decisions for their families and their children.

Karen and her husband, Bill, have two boys, Eric (twenty-one) and John (nineteen), both of whom are on the autism spectrum and were diagnosed in elementary school. Karen's boys are a prime example of the fact that autism manifests differently in each individual—even within the same family. Eric was hyper-alert with attention challenges, while John displayed social immaturity and **food jags**. Both boys are highly functional and now successful in college. They are active members of their church. Although both boys are very different from one another, their talents and challenges complement one another.

Sarah's son Mitchell was diagnosed late, at nine years old. She and her husband, Tom, also have a twelve-year-old daughter with anxiety and an adopted seven-year-old son from South Korea. Mitchell (thirteen) struggles with social pragmatics and executive functioning skills, but was accelerated a grade level in school and is fascinated by deep science, amphibians and reptiles, and complicated math algorithms.

THE ROUND TABLE QUESTIONS

Here are the questions I posed that evening:

- Describe one or two behaviors related to your child's autism that you find endearing.
- Does autism consume and define your family?
- How has your child's autism shaped the character of their sibling(s)?
- If you could go back in time, what would you tell yourself immediately following your child's diagnosis?
- Tell me a story you'll never forget related to your child's autism.
- Besides yourself, who has made the biggest impact on your child and how?

timeline

The timeline shows key dates including significant milestones, therapies, doctors' appointments, and diagnoses in order to more easily track Hannah's journey. While it will help you follow our story, keep in mind that every child with autism is different and develops at his or her own rate.

February 2005   Hannah is born.

April 2006   Hannah contracts an upper respiratory infection, croup, and bilateral ear infections.

May 2006   Hannah is having trouble transitioning to table food, not talking or babbling, and is no longer pulling up on objects. Pediatrician recommends state's early intervention services and a consultation with a pediatric neurologist. He believes Hannah has one of three possible **pervasive developmental disorders (PDD)**.

June 2006   Hannah passes her hearing test. She begins physical therapy and occupational therapy provided by our state's early intervention services.

July 2006	My husband and I find out we're expecting our second child, Connor. Hannah begins speech therapy and developmental therapy through the state's early intervention services.
August 2006	A visit to the pediatric neurologist designates Hannah's preliminary diagnosis of autism. We choose to seek an official diagnosis. The pediatric neurologist refers Hannah to a developmental pediatrician and a behavioral psychologist for an official diagnosis of autism.
October 2006	Hannah visits the orthopedist to be fitted for her Suresteps.
November 2006	Hannah has her first visit with the developmental pediatrician who orders an MRI of her brain and spine. The developmental pediatrician refers Hannah to a gastroenterologist and dietitian. Hannah begins to walk.
January 2007	Hannah sees a gastroenterologist and dietitian for the first time. The gastroenterologist orders a swallow/feeding study.
February 2007	A behavioral psychologist gives Hannah her first official diagnosis of autism. Hannah has an MRI that reveals no medical anomalies of the brain or spine.
March 2007	Hannah has a swallow/feeding study that shows no anatomical obstructions that would lead to severe food aversions. Connor is born.
April 2007	Hannah begins feeding therapy.

May 2007	Hannah begins behavioral therapy.
June 2007	Hannah receives her second official diagnosis of autism.
February 2008	Hannah enters developmental preschool.
May 2008	Hannah is able to articulate approximately ten words. She begins aquatic therapy.
June 2008	Hannah begins social/play therapy.
August 2008	Hannah adds Play-N-Share Preschool to her schedule.
August 2009	Hannah adds Light and Life Preschool to her schedule.
April 2010	Hannah begins equine-assisted therapy.
November 2012	Hannah's autism diagnosis is more specifically characterized as Asperger's syndrome.
June 2015	Hannah begins work with what she calls her life coach (a different behavioral management specialist).

CHAPTER ONE
the "d" word

Diagnosis/Identification

Autism is part of my child. It's not everything he is. My child is so much more than a diagnosis.

—S. L. Coelho

June 2007

*I'm on summer break from school and home with the kids—where I want to be. Hannah is out on the swing set with her occupational therapist for **sensory modulation** before her therapy session officially begins. Back in February we received by letter an official diagnosis of autism from the behavioral psychologist, but I didn't want to believe it. In late May we went to the Autism Treatment Center for a second opinion. On this lazy June afternoon, while Hannah is safe with the therapist and Connor is napping in his Pack 'n Play, I head to the front of the house and open the mailbox. It's the letter. I'm not sure why it takes me a while to open the envelope of the letter that I've been waiting to receive.*

The doctor at the Autism Treatment Center seemed hesitant to tell us anything about his findings in person; we had to wait for this letter. I finally tear open the envelope and scan the first page. Looks like he accurately documented our chief concerns and Hannah's history. I turn to the second page.

The typed words make me sick. Angry. Who the hell does this doctor think he is? The family history, social history, and mental status examination sections read: "The mother has a Master's Degree and denies a history of mental health problems or substance abuse on her side of the family. Father has a Master's Degree as well, but his mother was adopted. So, there is little known about his family history. However, to father's knowledge, he denies any history of mental health problems or substance abuse on his side of the family. Parents have made sure their daughter was clean, and her hair was combed. Hannah also wore attire that was appropriate for age and weather."

We were there for an autism evaluation. Why does it matter whether or not we have college degrees? Are they suggesting that substance abuse caused Hannah's autism? The worst substance I have ever consumed was alcohol, and I never did that when I was pregnant with either of my children. Why would my daughter not be clean? Why wouldn't I comb her hair? I'm so mad I can hardly concentrate, but finally I see it—the "D" word. At the bottom of the page: Our second official diagnosis of autism.

I pushed my baby girl's stroller into the doctor's office for her fifteen-month checkup with our pediatrician on May 25th. I would have carried her, but she really disliked being touched. After a full day of teaching, I picked her up from daycare and drove straight to the doctor's office. To this day, I wish I'd asked my husband to go with me, but I didn't. I went alone. Hannah had recently lost a few skills she had developed. She didn't make much eye contact these days and wasn't even watching those around her. Smiles were rare. Her toddler developmental toys confused her, and she wasn't imitating actions performed by others. She would focus on ceiling fans indefinitely if allowed, and would line up her blocks instead of stacking them. I thought it was a setback from an upper respiratory infection she had a month prior, so I planned to discuss that with the doctor.

During her appointment, as the pediatrician worked through a milestone checklist, I thought, "This is not going well." On his notes from our last visit, before the respiratory infection, he had documented that Hannah was beginning to pull up. She was no longer doing that. He asked about babbling and putting things into her mouth. I answered she was not babbling yet at all and had never put anything into her mouth.

I explained that she seemed sensitive to the texture of foods and was having a terrible time transitioning to table foods. She was still primarily eating lower-stage baby food, yogurt, applesauce, and rice cereal. During our visit, Hannah became agitated and began flapping her hands. My husband and I always believed this was the way Hannah showed her excitement. We later learned this was an autistic trait for **self-regulation** known as stimming. Hannah would flap her arms as an expression of excitement or to calm herself.

Before this visit, the doctor assured us Hannah would meet her milestones in her own time—she wasn't in a hurry, he said, because she didn't have older siblings to keep up with. The May 25 visit was different. With uncharacteristic sternness, Dr. McIntire said he believed Hannah had one of three possible **pervasive developmental disorders**, a developmental delay.

I was shell-shocked. My baby, delayed? And what did "pervasive" mean? He pulled out a sheet of paper and scribbled the three diagnoses he wanted to explore with Hannah: **Pervasive Developmental Disorder—Not Otherwise Specified**, autism, and **Rett syndrome**. My heart seemed to stop pumping, and each breath felt strained. I did my best to be strong and hear every word this man said, but I had trouble concentrating. I blinked back tears that blurred my vision and kept my hands on Hannah's shoulders, to steady her on the exam table . . . to steady myself. How could I recover from the blow and retain information at the same time?

He discussed the therapies provided by the state of Indiana: physical therapy, occupational therapy, speech therapy, and developmental therapy. I was listening, but this was too much information, coming way too fast. He advised me to have Hannah evaluated for physical and occupational therapy through First Steps, Indiana's early intervention program. The recommendation of physical therapy was due to Hannah's low muscle tone and lack of gross motor skills. Sensory processing disorder, formerly sensory integration dysfunction, could play a role in developmental delays—a good therapist could explain the different sensory systems and determine Hannah's hyper- or hyposensitivity to each. Hannah's sensory input—the way she would take in information from the environment—was getting in the way of typical development. A child with autism often either over-responds or under-responds to sensory input. That would be the occupational therapist's main area of focus.

Dr. McIntire's nurse and secretary stepped into the room to walk me through the First Steps intake paperwork and the instructions for getting my daughter the help she needed, but they also tried to calm me with small gestures of compassion. One put a hand on my back as she explained the focus of the two therapies the doctor suggested. His secretary occupied Hannah as I clearly struggled to process everything. Their kindness took the edge off the panic I could feel shooting through me. I looked at Hannah and ran my hand down her little overalls to smooth them and settle her fidgety legs, hoping the gesture might calm my shaking hands at the same time. She was getting loud and restless.

Their kindness helped, but I kept thinking, "I need my husband." My husband was not only the love of my life and confidant, he had always been a source of great strength. As the medical staff threw all of this information at me, I needed him as a sounding board. This was not happening to us!

Dr. McIntire explained the urgency of getting in to see the neurologist as soon as possible to accurately diagnose or rule out Rett syndrome as our biggest fear. Of the three diagnoses he was leaning toward, only Rett syndrome included the lack of gross motor skills—walking—as an attribute. He would send all of our information to the neurologist's office, and I was to call the next day to set an appointment. By this point we'd been there so long, Hannah needed a break. I scooped up my little girl and placed her in the stroller to leave.

As I walked out the doors, I wasn't the same woman who walked in an hour earlier. I'd never be the same again. And I would always see Hannah differently.

I waited until I was in my car with Hannah safely clicked into her car seat before releasing the tears. After I controlled the heaving sobs and cleaned up my face with a wad of napkins I found in the glove compartment, I picked up the phone to call my husband. I then realized I wasn't ready to tell him. Not over the phone. Not while he was at work. He needed to hear the doctor's preliminary diagnosis in person. So I called my best friend, who is also one of my teaching partners: Lori, my voice of reason. And yes, we share the same name.

She was almost as shocked as I was with the information, as there was an atypical silence on the other end of the phone. She promised to come with us to the neurology appointment and do anything we needed. While that was comforting, it didn't change Dr. McIntire's words.

When my husband came home that evening from work, I shared the diagnosis. He said that he, like the pediatrician, believed that Hannah could be developmentally delayed. His matter-of-fact response confused me—to me, the phrase "developmental delay" sounded harsh and hopeless, like a permanent condition with no chance of "catching up." How could he take it so lightly? I felt a little scorned and needed to protect the sanctity of the little girl I pushed into the doctor's office.

The next day at school, I pulled aside my two teaching partners, Lori and Janet, and continued to share my fears. I told them about my husband's response—how he agreed with the doctor that Hannah must be developmentally delayed. I was still really upset that he thought it could be a possibility. They explained that the phrase "developmentally delayed" did not mean she wouldn't eventually reach the milestones—it would just take her more work and longer to reach them. They assured me when Hannah reached the same grade as the students we teach—sixth grade—she would probably already be caught up. Maybe even before then. As mothers, they were able to comfort me and offer hope that made sense. During our conversation, we had retreated to the restroom for more privacy. I was able to clean myself up and pull myself together because of their words.

I called the neurologist's office on my lunch break that day—they said it would be six months before his secretary could get us in.

No way. That was too long to wait for answers. I immediately called our pediatrician's office to see if they could get us in sooner. The following Monday they told me to call the neurologist back and try to schedule. Sure enough, the neurologist's office was going to work us in. Five weeks later, during our summer vacation, we were in.

SIGNS OF AUTISM[1]

- May avoid eye contact
- May prefer to be alone
- Echoes words or phrases
- Difficulty interacting with others
- Spins objects or self
- Insistence on sameness
- Inappropriate laughing or giggling
- Inappropriate attachments to objects
- May not want cuddling
- Difficulty in expressing needs; may use gestures
- Inappropriate response or no response to sound
- No real fear of dangers
- Apparent insensitivity to pain
- Sustained, unusual, or repetitive play; uneven physical or verbal skills

SIGNS OF SENSORY PROCESSING DISORDER[2]

- Extra sensitive to touch
- Sensitivity to sounds
- Picky eaters
- Avoidance of sensory stimulation
- Uneasiness with movement
- Hyperactivity
- Fear of crowds
- Poor fine or gross motor skills
- Excessive risk-taking
- Trouble with balance

THE FIRST VISIT

The office was small for a renowned neurologist. I felt the surroundings smothering and the building dated. As promised, my friend Lori came along to take care of Hannah and listen to the neurologist's answers to the questions I planned to ask. I knew I'd struggle to retain everything on my own, so if she took notes, my husband and I would be free to focus during the appointment and could study the information in more detail later.

I remember looking at the kids in his waiting room. Did they, too, have special needs? What were their diagnoses? I glanced at the parents and wondered if they were thinking the same exact same thing about my child.

The nurse called Hannah's name and led us to an exam room. The obligatory blood pressure cuff and scale created a challenge, given Hannah's sensory challenges and inability to stand on her own. The nurse didn't ask many questions, but the doctor did. As I learned after appointments with specialists of all kinds, the parents' introductory visit always begins with a history from the very beginning—pregnancy. Then a long list of questions makes the mother feel responsible for her child's diagnosis. And the self-inflicted guilt hurts when it shouldn't even be considered.

As the nurse closed the door behind her, I saw the following signs posted on the back of the door: 14 SIGNS OF AUTISM, AUTISM SCREENING, and WHY DOES MY KID DO THAT? 10 COMMON SIGNS OF SENSORY PROCESSING DISORDER. Yes, I knew right then. The neurologist's posters confirmed what I found when I did my own research. Hannah had autism. I swallowed hard, trying to force down the lump rising in my throat.

I knew, but I still needed to hear it from someone else, someone official.

The neurologist, Dr. Pappas, concentrated on Hannah and her behaviors the entire visit. This impressed me. He took copious notes and spoke into an old-fashioned mini-recorder. His demeanor was like that of a professor, but he handled Hannah like a seasoned dad. I had no doubts about his knowledge, warmth, or experience. After listening to our concerns, watching Hannah's behaviors, looking at our pediatrician's notes, and giving Hannah a physical examination, he concluded that Hannah did have autism. It felt official. He said we would have to see a behavioral psychologist through First Steps or arrange an appointment through the Christian Sarkine Autism Treatment Center at Riley Children's Hospital to get a formal evaluation and diagnosis, but he was sure. So, this was only another preliminary diagnosis? Maybe one of the behavioral psychologists would have something different to say.

He said to contact the Christian Sarkine Autism Treatment Center right away because sometimes families face a two-year wait for an evaluation. That didn't seem very promising. Or acceptable. I felt control over my daughter's plight slipping away visit by visit.

Now it was time for our questions:

What is a pervasive developmental disorder?

Answer: A group of five disorders, all characterized by delays in socialization and communication.

Can girls have autism?

Yes.

We thought it was more likely for boys?

Correct.

Is there a brain scan that can be done to test for autism?

No, but a brain scan could rule out other causes for delays.

Does Hannah have Rett syndrome, and how will you test for this?

This answer was more involved. He explained that Rett syndrome is a neurodevelopmental disorder that affects girls almost exclusively, characterized by normal early growth and development followed by a slowing of development, loss of purposeful use of the hands, distinctive hand movements, slowed brain and head growth, problems with walking, seizures, and intellectual disability.

He described some characteristics of Rett syndrome, like hand wringing, which I had seen Hannah do before, failure to want to eat and lack of chewing, loss of eye contact, and a loss of skills—all of which Hannah was exhibiting. I glanced over at Hannah. She wasn't wringing her hands at that moment. Oh, Lord, did she have Rett syndrome?

Rett syndrome shows up in one out of 10,000–15,000 girls. Those odds still didn't make me feel better. He said Hannah's normal head size and the fact that she wasn't wringing her hands while she was in his office were good signs. She probably didn't have Rett syndrome, but they had to perform the testing anyway, to rule it out.

Halfway through this rough question and answer exchange, Lori nudged me. "You're asking the questions, but not truly listening to his answers." Lori was doing her best to calm Hannah, who was growing agitated, and take notes for me at the same time. I nodded. I knew she was taking notes, and I was overwhelmed. Working my way through these questions kept me from collapsing—plus, I wanted to fit them all in before the appointment was over, so I was barreling through. I trusted Lori to take detailed notes I could look back on, but she was right. I had to focus on this information myself. I needed to stay strong and concentrate.

Dr. Pappas explained the tests: genetic blood testing and metabolic testing using blood and urine. He used lab names such as complete metabolic panel, thyroid testing, urine genetics screening, cytogenics chromosomal study, subtelomeric fish study, lactic acid study, and Rett DNA sequencing study. None of these could be done in his office. He would also be sending us to a developmental pediatrician to further help Hannah with other challenges such as walking, feeding, and gastrointestinal issues.

I asked two more questions: "Will Hannah ever catch up to her peers?" and "Will Hannah ever be mainstreamed into a general education classroom?" We had to know. After all, we weren't only her parents—we were both full-time educators.

He answered with a soft, compassionate, simple "No." Given the problems Hannah was currently having and the regression of her skills, he did not think she would be mainstreamed into a general education, grade-level-appropriate classroom with typical peers. He believed Hannah's needs would best be served in the future in a self-contained Life Skills class.

PROCESSING THE FIRST DAY

The three of us—Lori, my husband, and I—left his office devastated. We would return home with a list of specialty doctors to see, blood tests to be drawn, urine to be collected, and, of course, insurance to be contacted. A few days earlier I had found out I was pregnant, and now we faced implications that autism could be genetic. Lori was not aware of my pregnancy until the appointment with Dr. Pappas.

All the way down the hall, to the elevator, and through the parking garage, none of us spoke a word. As we got into the car, Lori realized we had forgotten to get a urine bag from the nurse to collect the specimen. The beginning of so many things to remember. We dropped her off in front of the office, and she ran in and got one. When Lori returned and sat in the front, I stayed in the back seat near Hannah. I could not stop looking at her as she was "in her own world."

After dropping Lori off at her house, we finally arrived home. I could see the news of autism was a heavy blow to my husband. Though he had easily taken the news that his daughter was developmentally delayed, he reacted much differently to the diagnosis of autism. I waited a moment before putting Hannah in her crib for a nap. He needed me. He headed straight to the couch and said, "How are we ever going to tell our friends and family Hannah has autism? I am so embarrassed."

He cried as he sank down into our couch in devastation. I patted Hannah's back and thought, "We are now different. We are now one of those families. My husband just confirmed it."

In Hannah's room, as I took off her shoes and settled her in her crib, I felt as though I had let my husband down. I did not give him the child he had wanted. He felt ashamed. As the mom, I thought I needed to "fix" the situation, so I resolved we could not both break down at the same time. I had to do everything in my power to help our daughter—not just for her, but for him, too. No, for all of us. And I resolved that day to get to know Hannah for her true self—not for the child we once thought she was. I was going to throw myself all into this, while I wasn't sure my husband would be able to wrap his head around it. Somehow, I was going to make this all okay for him.

MORE THAN A MOM: MY NEW JOB

Obtaining the urine and blood samples turned into a project. I was unable to collect a sample from Hannah at home, as she could not articulate her need to use the restroom. So, our pediatrician reluctantly agreed to catheterize Hannah, knowing how terrifying this would be for her. She had to lie on her back in the doctor's office and have a tube placed into her. He kept shaking his head, but there was no other way. I held her down while she tried to thrash and flail her arms and legs—her trauma ramped up due to her touch sensitivity.

Of course the doctor's office that performed her catheterization was not the one the neurologist wanted to handle her blood draw. So I had to drive all the way downtown to another facility. I've heard mothers talk about how they leave the room for their children's immunizations so their child won't witness them present during their pain. I've never had that luxury. With Hannah's sensory processing disorder and upper respiratory infection, I learned how to hold Hannah so the medical professionals could get their job done quickly and minimize trauma to my daughter. I would place her in my lap with her back at my chest. My left arm would then pin down her arms, and her legs could kick without touching anyone. My right hand was then free to either wipe her tears or hold her hair back. I used this same holding technique when brushing her teeth.

Hannah's father was rarely able to go to these appointments because of his demanding job, so I was left alone to locate all of the different hospitals and doctors' offices, navigate their parking garages, and fill out loads of intake paperwork. This was before insurance approved autism as a diagnosis, so most of these visits were out of pocket.

The deterioration rate, quality of life, and life expectancy for children with Rett syndrome are grim. The testing was supposed to take three months, and it ended up taking five. Fearful and bold, I phoned the triage nurse at the neurologist's office once a week to check if results were in. At the end of the fifth month of waiting, she called me at school with the best Christmas present ever: Hannah's genetic tests were negative for Rett syndrome. I've kept the paperwork to this day.

Hannah didn't have Rett syndrome, but she did have autism. In addition to the neurologist's verbal diagnosis, we were given official diagnoses from two other doctors. The first came from First Steps. First Steps had a behavioral psychologist come to our home and Hannah's daycare, observing Hannah at length in both locations. I could tell this medical professional had years of practical experience with children and parents. She recognized Hannah's autism right away and wasn't afraid to give us a play-by-play account of identification, the triggers (antecedents) that could be causing some of the behaviors, and several strategies to put into place to overcome her challenges. She was intrigued with Hannah lining up her flashcards, repeatedly pressing the same button on the same toy over and over again, not turning her head when her name was called, army crawling at her age, no eye contact, a disconnected look, lack of feeding skills, flapping, and a variety of other traits.

We received her formal diagnosis and verification in the mail one month later. Though the psychologist's demeanor had been positive in tone, the letter of formal diagnosis and the given conclusive data hurt. Her one letter actually felt like a life sentence, as it was the first time that I had official paperwork that spelled out in black and white that my daughter's life would be most challenging.

The second diagnosis came from Riley Children's Hospital's Christian Sarkine Autism Treatment Center. We had been told that we would wait approximately fifteen to eighteen months for an appointment. Fortunately, we were able to see a specialist in less than six months.

Hannah was fussy that day. I thought we were going to see the doctor in charge of the center; instead, a psychologist sat down with the three of us and said he would be doing the evaluation. Once again, we answered all the intake questions that are so painful for the mother.

He asked the standard list of questions such as:

- Did you conceive naturally?
- Did you contract any illnesses during your pregnancy?
- Did you take any drugs during your pregnancy?
- Did you smoke during your pregnancy?
- Did you drink any alcohol while pregnant?
- Did you exercise during pregnancy?
- What kind of exercise did you do and how often?
- Did you take prenatal vitamins during your pregnancy?
- How much weight did you gain during your pregnancy?

- Did you have gestational diabetes during pregnancy?
- Did you have any accidents during your pregnancy?
- Did your pregnancy go full term?
- Was there anything unusual about labor and delivery?
- Is there any lead paint in your home?
- Have immunizations been done routinely?
- Is there a history of autism in either of your families?

No wonder most mothers worry about maternal misgivings. As the man worked his way down the list, I felt I was being judged by him and my husband. I know that was only my perception—after all, maybe the questions are driven by autism research as they search for its cause—but I couldn't help feeling scrutinized. Was I the culprit? Since then, I have become familiar with Dr. Alycia Halladay at the Autism Science Foundation. Alycia is the foundation's chief science officer, and her foundation is studying the brains of individuals who had autism during their life in order to see which structures and functions are altered. Check them out at TakesBRAINS.org.

For the record, I didn't smoke, drink alcohol, take any type of drugs, have any illnesses, have any history of autism on either side of our families that we were aware of, or have lead paint in our home.

After observing Hannah for a while, interviewing us, and looking at the intake questionnaires, behavioral assessments, sensory profiles, and all the previous doctors' notes, he ended our meeting and said the summary with conclusion would be mailed within the following month.

One June afternoon, I got the mail and found the letter. After a few moments, I ripped it open, skimmed the long summary of diagnosis that categorically went over the diagnostic criteria. It cited clear evidence that without a doubt, Hannah had autism. The summary said that Hannah's intact family was a strength for her.

Our daughter had autism. We mourned, and I had to share the information with our parents. My husband's father responded, "How does that make you feel?" It felt like those words knocked the wind out of me. They kicked me when I was already down, but I had to focus on moving forward.

⚬⚭⚮ **Wisdom from the Round Table** ⚬⚭⚮

Lori R.: There is hope after a diagnosis. Hope for the best life possible for your family. Hope to dream new dreams for your child. Hope that they will be loved and embraced by others. The list goes on. Hope is a powerful thing.

Jen: Noah is not autistic; he has autism. It's not something he asked to be given. It's the way God designed him.

Lori V.: A diagnosis of autism allowed Byron an IEP at school. The IEP and the school system's autism consultant were of great benefit for Byron. I knew I needed to advocate for my son in order for him to have the tools he needed.

Susan: Our families have never thought of us as anything other than good parents. There was no blame, no shunning, no excluding Tyler from things, and no thinking they could do a better job.

Karen: Eric was first diagnosed with attention deficit hyperactivity disorder (ADHD) only. I felt there was not enough behavioral help. A teacher then identified his autism, and I felt there was much more support.

Sarah: Now that Mitchell has a diagnosis, his behaviors make sense for the first time in his life. Now I can work to help him, and it's no longer a fight against it. Now we know what we need to do.

CHAPTER TWO

life before autism

Being a mother is learning about strengths you didn't know you had, and dealing with fears you didn't know existed.

—Linda Wooten

February 2005

Today is the day we've eagerly anticipated for nine months—the birth of our daughter, Hannah Grace. My obstetrician has chosen to induce my labor due to my recent stress test results and gestational diabetes. I've even had the luxury of being off work and on bed rest this past week.

As we walk through the atrium to the admissions desk, today feels like no other. Our daughter will be a combination of everything we've done that is good. The two of us are planners, so we've attended every evening class provided by the hospital from Lamaze to Safety for Your Newborn. This place will always feel extraordinary, almost sacred, to us.

Check-in goes smoothly, and we're excited to hear that a suite is available after the delivery—a relief, as suites can't be reserved. After securing our wristbands, the admissions clerk escorts us into the eleva-tor, which takes us to the labor and delivery section of the hospital. We stop at the nurses' station and meet Cindy, our labor and deliv-ery nurse. Cindy's demeanor seems soft, charitable, and kindhearted. Immediately I sense she's a caretaker. She walks us to our assigned room—*all the way at the end of a long hallway.* Looks like they could have placed us closer to the nurses' station.

Sounds from across the hallway reveal that someone's bundle of joy has already arrived. Our anticipation is escalating. Cindy hands me two plastic bags with the hospital's name and emblem to store my clothes. She instructs me to slip into the light blue hospital gown. I need to save the bags as mementoes from my daughter's birth.

I lie down in the bed, and Cindy begins my intake evaluation after making sure I'm covered and comfortable. We find out we both live in the same suburb west of the city. Then, as luck would have it, we discover her daughter attends the school where I teach. I think about the ramifications—how embarrassing!

She attaches a heart monitor for my baby and contacts my obstetrician, Dr. Allen, to let him know I'm ready. He arrives chipper and, like always, wearing a bow tie. He examines me and finds I'm not dilated any more than last week in his office. He says there's no way to accurately project how long it's going to take for the Pitocin to trigger the dilation and contractions to occur. He explains that when the time is right, Cindy will contact him to order the epidural. Cindy begins to administer the Pitocin via IV around 9:30.

At noon, Cindy reports to Dr. Allen that dilation is moving very slowly, so he increases the Pitocin dosage. My parents arrive around this time, and we're glad to have company. I am now in a pleasant, even dreamy, mood because Dr. Allen also ordered Nubain for pain relief. When is my little girl going to enter this world?

Dr. Allen pops back in around 3:00 and short introductions are made to my parents. This is only after he knocks first, and my dad answers with, "Nobody's home." Dad! How embarrassing! *My parents leave the room and remark that the next time they see us, I'll have Hannah in my arms. Good thoughts! The doctor examines me and decides to go ahead and break my water manually. Apparently my little girl is happy right where she is and needs a little encouragement to come out into the world.*

The anesthesiologist arrives at 3:45 to administer the epidural. As the needle enters my spine, I feel a sharp pain. I grip my husband's hand for dear life. The epidural is worse than I thought it would be. I'm sure it will be worth it.

Cindy's shift is over at 4:00, and she hands me over to Maggie. Nurse Maggie has to be in her late sixties and is already barking orders like a drill sergeant. Things aren't set up as she wants them. Nurse Maggie checks me again. "Where is the doctor?" she complains. "We're having this baby by 5:00." She pages Dr. Allen, and he's here within minutes. My doctor laughs, and explains that Maggie's been around for a very long time.

At 4:30 I start pushing. I push for over twenty minutes but Hannah makes no progress. Now Dr. Allen fears she'll go into distress if I don't deliver soon. Wanting to avert distress, he quickly performs an episiotomy.

Hannah Grace Taylor arrives at 4:57, weighing seven pounds and ten ounces. We're overwhelmed with happiness. She has a massive amount of jet-black hair and a dark complexion—like mine. Nurse Maggie uses an inkpad to place Hannah's footprints on a knit hat which she places on my husband's head—turns out she can be quite personable and humorous after all. Hannah is then swaddled in a blanket with burgundy, pink, light blue, and green footprints. Our perfect baby is placed into my arms.

Birth is a miracle. We've never known an overwhelming love like this. Time needs to stand still. Nothing can feel better than this moment. I look down at her perfect nose, her perfect lashes. I know the swell of a mother's heart and think, Hannah's needs will always come before ours.

I stare at her—can't take my eyes off her. I'm so blessed to call her mine. The future has so much in store for her.

Though you can never go back to the way things were, you can certainly look back. In fact, I believe it can be helpful to reflect on the "before" in order to appreciate the people and circumstances that helped orchestrate where you are today.

My husband and I were an idealistic couple with big dreams and goals for our future. We loved, supported, and respected one another, truly complementing each other in personality, skills, and interests. In the areas of family, finances, and careers, we usually had a plan and were cautious with our moves. However, we would also sweat the small, insignificant stuff, like keeping up with the Joneses. One day, we would learn the small stuff didn't matter one bit, but before . . . it did. And we would conclude that control is only an illusion. Some situations are beyond us. There's a life you dream of and the one you actually live.

MARRIAGE

We met as a result of teaching within the same school district. I had first spotted him at a back-to-school event in the fall of 2000. Towering at six feet, five inches, tall, thin, handsome—I couldn't help but notice his presence. I discreetly arranged for a middle school teacher to introduce the two of us. And it took off from there!

We exchanged emails and spoke on the phone. Later, I found out he'd printed and saved those emails, which meant a lot. He was twenty-seven, and I was thirty. He was originally from New York, and I was from Indiana. Our families and backgrounds were totally different, but we fit perfectly. He was a good listener, dependable, and caring—the reason I fell in love. He had lived a careful, cautious life, and I believe I forced him to step outside his comfort zone to enjoy some different things that life has to offer, like appreciating the ocean on a Wave Runner and exploring Hawaii's beauty from above during a helicopter excursion. We relished sharing teaching stories, going to Indianapolis Colts football games, watching movies, going out to eat, visiting our alma mater, Indiana University, and hiking in state parks.

We became inseparable and better because the other was there. We had a life. We had each other. We could confide our innermost thoughts with one another. Nothing could shake this foundation—we were sure of it. Our relationship was healthy and happy.

On a weekend sightseeing trip to Chicago in 2002, we took a carriage ride. He had the driver stop at a popular downtown square, held out a small box, and then proposed with a beautiful ring. We dined at a nice Italian restaurant, enjoyed a celebratory dessert, and returned to a hotel room with a vase of red roses.

We bought a house—the perfect place to start our family.

On our wedding day, my husband's profile against the church's stained-glass windows melted my heart. We recited our vows, exchanged rings, and celebrated with friends at a reception held at a yacht club that overlooked a reservoir. I married my best friend that day, and every moment was a testament of our love for one another. It was the happiest day of my life. Nothing could break this bond.

CAREERS

Our careers were important to our identity. We enjoyed our subject areas and our students. He was also a team leader and girls' basketball coach. It felt as if he was doing a lot of work and putting in a lot of time for what he was being paid.

Before we knew one another, he had begun his administrative license in education, and we both agreed that maybe it was time that he finished it. I also longed for continued education, but I already held a master's degree in curriculum and instruction. I decided that a license in gifted and talented and **twice-exceptional** (2e—the student is both gifted and has a learning, emotional, behavioral, or social challenge) education was the route I wanted to go. We helped one another out with our classwork. As a coach, he couldn't attend a few of his classes, so I gladly stepped in and took notes for him. He also helped me navigate the technology required for my online classes. In the meantime, we found comfort and support working in the same school system.

We methodically had begun to pile up one good thing after another without realizing that stretching one another too thin would upset the balance in our relationship. When we added the responsibility of providing the care our child would need, it quickly became evident that we had too much on our plates and our relationship suffered.

Know that just because something is a good thing doesn't mean that it's a good thing right now. In looking back, I wish I had taken my own advice.

A CHILD IS BORN

My husband and I both wanted to have children. I was a few years older than him, and I felt my biological clock ticking—especially if we wanted more than one child. We had trouble getting pregnant at first, so we went to a fertility specialist, who didn't put me on any fertility drugs but prescribed a medication to counteract a blood level that was not helping with fertility. Not long after going on the medication, I found out I was pregnant and could not wait to share the news with my husband.

School had just let out for the summer break. I asked my husband if we could go to a local park. I'd stopped at a bookstore the day before to purchase *What to Expect When You're Expecting* and found a comparable book for dads, *The Expectant Father*. I wrapped the book along with a baby's bib that read "I Love My Daddy" and handed the package to him. He unwrapped the book and the bib, read the card, and we knew our lives were going to change in the best possible way. A baby! This was exactly what we longed for.

During the pregnancy, my husband would join me at every doctor's appointment I deemed necessary. Before the ultrasound appointment, my doctor predicted we were having a little girl by listening to the heartbeat. The ultrasound confirmed it. We decided to call her Hannah Grace. I ate right, exercised, and got plenty of sleep, following the advice of *What to Expect When You're Expecting* and my doctor's input. I did develop gestational diabetes, but it didn't complicate my pregnancy as much as it could have.

Everything proceeded normally. My friends got giddy the more I started to show. A friend helped me register for my baby showers, where family and friends spoiled our family. We designed the dream nursery with murals to decorate the walls—butterflies and daisies. My grandmother's hand-sewn quilt adorned the finest designer crib. A matching bookshelf contained popular children's books—*The Very Hungry Caterpillar; Goodnight Moon; Corduroy; Brown Bear, Brown Bear, What Do You See?;* and more. A mobile hung over the crib dangling fuzzy pastel letter blocks overhead. We were ready for our little girl to arrive.

So many visitors showed up to welcome Hannah Grace into the world. I will never forget the heavenly two days we spent in the hospital. The nursing staff commented that Hannah was the only new-born in the nursery not wearing the hospital's garments. All of our visitors wrote words of good fortune on a picture mat. That mat with Hannah's name and birthdate in calligraphy would surround her new-born picture. My husband had my favorite flowers, Gerbera daisies, delivered to the hospital. We made sure we bought the day's newspapers: the *Indianapolis Star* and *USA Today*. Staff would come in at all hours to check on me. Breastfeeding was a challenge at first because Hannah kept falling asleep, so my husband tried to help wake her.

Like most first-time parents, we were apprehensive the day we left the hospital; however, we prepared Hannah by dressing her in a tiny onesie and a warm, white and pink button-up sweater with a flowered collar and matching pants. My husband asked the nurse if we could stay another day. My mother laughed because she thought he was just kidding, but I knew my husband was just scared. We managed to stall the nurses while we looked at the room one last time, for memory's sake. My husband was so nervous to drive Hannah home that he was actually swerving in each direction on the highway. I rode in the back seat with Hannah so I could gaze at her beautiful face, keep a hand on her car seat, and make sure she was fine.

I took six months off from my job to stay home with Hannah. Of course that included the two months of the summer when school was out anyway. That June my husband accepted his first assistant principal's job. It was a hard decision for him to make for several reasons. He really did like teaching, and the administrator's position was one hour and fifteen minutes from our home. Despite the long drive and the shift away from teaching, we decided it was advantageous for our family. The job would mean a better salary with paid benefits and gave him administrative experience—essential to my husband because he wanted to one day become an administrator in our current school system. We made the best choice we could at the time.

That one decision was probably the worst we would ever make in our relationship. We didn't know a storm was about to hit our family. We didn't realize my husband becoming an administrator so soon meant he would be far away in our time of need. We didn't know we would have a life before, and a life after. All we knew was life at that moment, as new parents deeply in love with each other and over the moon about our newborn baby girl. All we knew was that life was good.

HOW A DIAGNOSIS MOVES A PARENT FORWARD FROM THE PAST[3]

❖ An autism diagnosis forces parents to evaluate their child earlier for their gifts and challenges rather than when parents normally evaluate for other traits like intelligence and athleticism. An example would be a child at age three that can put a jigsaw puzzle together in no time but cannot utilize their words to describe simple events.

❖ An autism diagnosis forces parents to change their epistemological standpoint or their life orientation— parents must adjust their vision of how they believe their child will learn. This takes longer if the child with autism is a firstborn. Parents may not know what to expect or when to expect it.

❖ An autism diagnosis forces parents to redirect their dreams. Success is now measured differently and in smaller increments.

❖ An autism diagnosis forces parents to change their levels of satisfaction in life. Parents are no longer worried about the different food groups as long as their children will eat. What used to be important to parents is no longer on their radar.

❖ An autism diagnosis forces parents to learn early how to advocate or fight for their child in a way that brings them success and doesn't hinder them. What we advocate for really matters—accommodations and modifications for our child. We aren't fighting for our children to be on the All-Star team; instead, we fight for our children to look someone in the eyes when they're speaking to them, or we fight for them to not speak blunt words that are understood to be rude.

༄ **Wisdom from the Round Table** ༄

Lori R.: I can confidently say that my three other children wouldn't change a thing. They will also tell you that we are a better and closer family because of having Cameron. Somehow the subject of Cameron never driving came up, so we talked about the reasons why. Caleb said, "He won't have to worry about driving anyway because he'll always have brothers and a sister to take him wherever he wants to go."

Jen: I still question if I should have waited and spread out the immunizations. I feel we gave Noah too many immunizations at one time. He received immunizations at fifteen months, which I feel could've waited closer to the age of two. Also, no one ever mentioned that if Noah had a cold, runny nose, or hadn't been well we shouldn't immunize at that visit. His immune system would have been low. Parents shouldn't be pressured to give immunizations just because it's "time" at that particular visit.

Lori V.: Before the diagnosis, I imagined our family doing many vacations together and being a solid unit. I wanted to be the "Kool-Aid" mom with all of the kids hanging out. Well, there were no friends for Byron and vacations were very hard with one child on the spectrum and one as neurotypical. Vacations were more of a juggling act and weren't vacations for me so we became a "stay at home" family for the most part. I learned to find some joy in just being there for both of my boys, even though in very different capacities.

Susan: When one of your children is diagnosed with autism, it's a diagnosis for the entire family. Life is never the same again.

Karen: Before our boys were diagnosed, we found their peculiar sayings and actions to be a source of fun and joy in our family. Then, when we understood that many of these peculiarities were autism-based, we felt quite badly.

Sarah: Mitchell had always amazed us with his intelligence and wit, and confounded us with unexplainable social and emotional struggles. Before his diagnosis of autism, we were lost.

CHAPTER THREE

something's not quite right

Early Signs and Worries

Children with autism are colorful—they are often very beautiful and, like the rainbow, they stand out.

—Adele Devine

February 2006

We're excited to celebrate Hannah's first birthday with friends and family. Over a month of planning has gone into this joyous celebration.

Guests begin to arrive at Gymboree Play and Music. Gymboree programs are especially designed to help young children learn and develop as they play—also a great host for kids' parties. As greetings and hugs are exchanged, I can't help but count my blessings. These are good people who care about our family. Hannah will grow up with their children, attend school on the Northside, play team sports, ride in carpools, and enjoy numerous slumber parties.

The Gymboree instructor calls parents and children into a large circle to begin the party. Hannah quickly becomes fascinated with a Gymbo the Clown decal on the mat and is not willing to join the circle.

All the other kids are seated in front of their parents with their attention focused on the instructor. I pull Hannah toward me and then notice that none of the other children are seated in the W-sitting position, which is typical for Hannah. We begin by singing a song while shaking plastic maracas. I'm fortunate it doesn't last long because Hannah is still focused on Gymbo and has covered her ears to muffle the sounds that disturb her.

The song ends and a large multi-colored parachute is stretched over the mat. Parents are instructed to place their children into the center and shake the outside of the parachute. Hannah feels the breeze and hears the soft sounds of the nylon material—other kids giggle, but Hannah flaps her hands and rolls her eyes up and back as she does when she's excited. As we all walk in a circle to rotate the parachute, Hannah is the only child without enough upper body strength to stay upright. She topples over.

When the parachute fun is complete, the instructor comes out with a bubble blower that releases a plethora of small bubbles that drift over the entire area above the parachute and our kids. Children run and crawl across the nylon waving their hands and arms in the air to catch and pop the bubbles. Hannah chooses one bubble to follow at a time, perhaps out of curiosity, but not out of delight or glee. They give her no pleasure whatsoever. As a matter of fact, she does not want them to touch her skin at all. She's completely unaware that the other kids are behaving differently, but I'm not. After the group activities are complete, kids begin to walk or crawl on their hands and knees off the parachute—not one child is army crawling, as Hannah is.

While families disperse to different areas of the spacious play gym, I'm surprised to see that so many of the kids are doing things that Hannah's never done before. Some of them are placing the ball pit's plastic balls into their mouths. Ugh! I think of the germs they can be contracting at this time of the year. I'm relieved Hannah has never done anything like that. Then I notice all of the kids are pulling up on the ladder of the slide. Hannah has not shown any interest in doing this yet. My husband and I try to get her to crawl through an expandable tunnel, but she seems afraid of it. Both of us take turns peeking through *the tunnel trying to cajole her but to no avail. I saw one of those for sale up front. Maybe I should buy one? Let her get used to it at home? She's found a plastic set of shapes that interests her. She places all the red circles together, all the green triangles together, and all of the blue squares together. She then continues to line up each category in perfect vertical columns. She's started to do the same thing at home with her building blocks.*

As we gather in the small party room, I'm delighted to see that the kids enjoy the birthday hats, blowers, and floating pink and lavender balloons. Parents comment on the two birthday cakes I ordered that are shaped and decorated as birthday presents with pink and lavender polka dots—one chocolate and one white. I've made sure my girl has her own special cake so she can dig in with both hands without ruining an entire cake that's to be served.

I begin to stretch the elastic string under Hannah's chin to hold the birthday hat, and she cringes, grabs the string, and struggles to get it off. Dismayed, I decide I'll remove the hat after she blows out the candle. She doesn't really need a birthday hat.

I then place her #1 cake in front of her and light the candle. Kids gather around and take turns showing her how to blow it out as I continually relight it. Hannah isn't interested in trying to blow the candle out. Her eyes grow larger as the children jockey for the birthday girl's attention. We sing "Happy Birthday" and, luckily, this doesn't bother her. One of the older kids then blows the candle out, and I remove Hannah's party hat. Many try to get her to put her hands into the cake to taste its delicious sweetness and make a complete mess, but that's simply not my daughter. Her dad is able to put a few bites into her mouth with a fork, and that's going to have to be good enough.

I think everyone's had a good time, but now Hannah is on overload, and her Nana, my mother-in-law, takes her into a quiet room away from the hustle and bustle and rocks her. I wish she would have been able to open presents, but Hannah gets agitated so easily when others are around. She really didn't seem to be engaged with any of the other children this evening. I'm sure it will come with time. Probably at her second birthday.

For over a year, I missed numerous red flags signaling autism—as if it was invisible. Hannah exhibited many autistic traits in daily life and during major events and outings, but she was our first child and we weren't around enough other children before having Hannah or even during her first year to spot or add up the signs. There was no baseline for comparison. We didn't realize she was approaching early developmental stages without hitting typical milestones. She was just our little Hannah, on her own timetable, revealing her own distinct personality. We worked around her preferences and let her take her time. I incorrectly believed the early developmental stages to be more fluid—unaware of the telltale signs of autism.

The signs are obvious to me now, in retrospect, as hallmarks of autism. By the time Hannah turned a year old, she should have been showing new skills and abilities. For example, she should have gained sufficient upper body strength to hold herself upright, been capable of pulling up, and certainly moved past the army crawling stage. We knew she exhibited other traits but didn't know they had names and labels, nor that they were tied to autism. Things like no **joint attention, perseveration** on objects, noise sensitivity, apathy to others' actions, W-sitting position, flapping of hands, absence of eye contact, tactile sensitivity, no exploring objects with mouth, **proprioception** issues, categorizing and lining up objects, apathy toward food, inability to **motor plan,** and sensory overload when responding to the environment. Besides, a child can be displaying some of these red flags and not have autism. But Hannah? Her traits began to add up—the sheer quantity she manifested should have told us that something wasn't quite right. If we'd known more about the diagnosis—if we understood the basics of autism—we might have recognized the possibility sooner. In Hannah's case, the signs of autism did multiply; however, I don't believe it was a case of retrograde autism—as I now believe there were always signs.

Don't miss the signs like we did.

AUTISM SCREENER FOR CHILDREN
UNDER TWO YEARS OF AGE[4]

+ Inactive
+ Limp or floppy
+ Very little crying
+ Limited social response
+ Limited social smile or eye contact
+ Limited engagement/awareness of others
+ Irritable
+ Difficult to comfort
+ Comforted only by motion
+ Limp/stiff when held
+ Unusual sensitivity to environmental input such as touch, smell, vision, or sound
+ Difficulty communicating
+ Limited understanding and/or use of specific gestures

AUTISM SCREENER FOR CHILDREN
OVER TWO YEARS OF AGE[5]

+ Inconsistency in use of functional communication
+ Difficulty expressing wants or needs
+ High levels of distress over minor changes
+ Limited conversation skills
+ Significant time spent seeking sensory input
+ Slamming into objects/people
+ Wedging self in tight places
+ Spinning in circles
+ Decreased sensitivity to pain
+ Any regression or loss of language skills
+ Interacting with others only to meet a particular need
+ Focused and repetitive interests dominate play
+ Little creative and imaginative play
+ Intense difficulty in understanding social interaction and safety rules

- ❖ Greater understanding of visual information
- ❖ Self-injurious behavior
- ❖ Repetitive whole body movements
- ❖ Repetitive movement of objects/toys

THE DOMINOES BEGIN TO FALL

We may have missed the signs, but eventually enough issues arose, one after another, that it became obvious she was different and might need some kind of help. The behaviors that stood out to us were her need for solitude to find comfort, her gastrointestinal issues, her inability to play like or with her peers, feeding and bathing challenges, lack of joint attention, and regression in several developmental areas.

COMFORT IN SOLITUDE

Hannah continued to grow, but she was a fussy baby. When offered a pacifier, she would spit it back out. I remember at one point in the summer of her first year reading the book *The Happiest Baby on the Block*, by Harvey Karp, MD. I read the book in a few hours, highlighting possible solutions, and I immediately tried the methods proposed to calm her. Nothing worked. I returned once more to her beloved bouncy seat. Hannah truly found comfort in it, and I relied on it. That seat was so integral to our sanity and her peace, I saved it; the seat is stored in my attic to this day. She could only tolerate being held about ten minutes at a time. As a first-time mother, I didn't know this was abnormal. As long as she was nestled in her seat, not held or forced to engage, she was truly satisfied. I had to resign myself that my little girl preferred no cuddling. Had I let her, she would have stayed in her bouncy seat all day without fussing a bit. She was also completely calmed and mesmerized by her Baby Einstein videos such as Baby Bach, Baby Mozart, Baby Newton, and Baby Van Gogh. She even smiled when anticipating the beginning of a new show, continually flapping her arms and bouncing her seat. All she had to hear was the introduction music. She truly felt a connection with the videos. What a shock to find out later that all four of those famous people had autism!

Hannah nursed fine and slept in a bassinet by our bed for the first three months. Before long, though, I was pumping, and she was outgrowing her bassinet. We moved her across the hallway to her crib. She was perfectly satisfied and content alone in her room. When she woke in the morning, she would occupy herself until we were ready to get her up to feed and bathe her, never trying to awaken us or pull up on the crib to get out.

GASTROINTESTINAL SIGNALS

I felt so happy to be back to work in the fall. I dropped off six-month-old Hannah at daycare that first day and drove to our school system's new intermediate building. Within a few hours, I received a call from the daycare. Something was already wrong. Hannah was constipated, unable to find relief. This had never happened before. My baby was experiencing pain, and I wasn't there when she needed me the most. That tore me apart. Thankfully, our daycare was only five minutes away, and I was able break away on that first day of school to go over and try to help. Little did I know at the time, but this was just the beginning of Hannah's gastrointestinal problems. Before Hannah was diagnosed with autism, I had no idea that many children with autism often have gastrointestinal difficulties.

PLAY

During Hannah's first year, we became members of Gymboree Play and Music and our local children's museum and zoo. At Gymboree we noticed that the other children seemed more alert to what was happening. Hannah seemed content doing her own thing at her own pace. Other behaviors that we found endearing in our home began to stand out as different or atypical in public. We also noticed that some of the children were babbling—a few were even saying words. Hannah was not doing this yet. Trips to the children's museum ended up stressful and draining as we slowly began to discover we were forcing Hannah to participate in a world that was extremely uncomfortable to her.

Pay attention to your child's responses to new situations. Touching the sand in the sand table, for Hannah, caused sensory overload, and after several visits we saw how excruciating it was for her compared with the kids around her. While others her age made their way through the plastic foam maze, she just sat on the comfortable foam mat and gazed into space. In another area, we would always find children placing colorful stemmed flowers into the holes where they belonged—a great fine motor activity. Hannah, however, had no idea how the holes were to be used. Trying to redirect her didn't help at all. Though it took us much longer than it should have, we eventually saw it: Hannah responded differently to the world than other children. When it came to play, she struggled to be present in our world and to us. Whether we were by her or in another room, she always seemed as if she were alone and content to be just that.

FEEDING

Feeding became a challenge for Hannah. She transitioned from milk to rice cereal perfectly. Stage-one and stage-two baby food transitions also went well. After that, she stopped transitioning. Stage-three foods like vegetable and turkey dinner and chicken noodle dinner had too much texture for Hannah. Food became an aversion. She never wanted to pick up table food because she would have to touch it. Trying to feed her a Cheerio or a cereal snack called Puffs always set off a major cry of panic and alarm. She simply didn't care for food, and at times seemed afraid of it. She had an instant gag reflex with projectile vomiting, so we usually just stuck with applesauce, stage-one and -two food, mashed potatoes, macaroni and cheese, and some stage-three foods. Every once in a while I'd accidentally drop a bit of cereal, baby food, yogurt, or applesauce on her and she would cry and flap her hands.

I'd watch other children when we went out to eat. They were either eating plate food, or chewing on Cheerios, crackers, or Puffs—and when a tiny dribble of food landed on them, they didn't shriek. I couldn't believe they weren't choking. They also seemed so strong sitting up in their high chairs. Hannah was still slouching, showing little upper body strength. The other kids were also coloring on their children's menu. Hannah hadn't shown any interest at all in doing this and seemed to be the same age. I remember feeling confused—but not worried. It would come with time, right?

BATHING

Drying Hannah off after a bath, combing her hair, brushing her teeth, and trimming her nails distressed her sensory nerves, and her obvious painful reactions to these everyday ablutions made me feel hopeless and worn out.

JOINT ATTENTION

At fourteen months old, Hannah wasn't yet turning to people when they said her name. Most of the time I felt like she was either in her own world or expressing frustration and panic. We'd see little kids her age wave at people. Hannah would wave with her palm facing herself if she would even try to wave at all. I learned later she was uncertain where her body was in space; in retrospect, that would explain her awkward movements and the disconnect between a movement and her intention.

She didn't seem to learn from watching others. I tried to teach her to clap and pat-a-cake, but she wouldn't try. She also wasn't pointing to objects in order to get our attention, though other kids her age did that all the time. I remember the Easter after Hannah turned one. Her cousin, Peyton, only four months older than Hannah, walked around the yard collecting Easter eggs in her basket. Hannah couldn't walk and had no idea she was supposed to be collecting eggs. She just sat in the grass staring with a glazed, unhappy look while Peyton brought the eggs to Hannah. She was *not there*.

REGRESSION

At this time, Hannah came down with a horrible upper respiratory infection, croup, and bilateral ear infections. She was inconsolable. I was supposed to take her down to my parents that weekend for a visit, but it would be over a three-hour drive. Should I go? I convinced myself to try. We headed out and she was crying so hard I considered turning around but continued on because we were at the halfway point.

When I arrived at my parents', we decided to take her to one of the convenient care-type medical offices. The young doctor reached out to introduce himself and gently touched Hannah, but she wouldn't allow him to make contact. She squirmed and wiggled and writhed at anything he said or did. He seemed shocked by her response. Her response wasn't new to me—Hannah had always been like this. The doctor was even more shocked when Hannah would not allow him to place the oscilloscope into her ear to check for ear infections. Didn't all kids behave like this? His odd scrutiny bewildered me. I'm sure people in the waiting room could hear her complete meltdown—shrill shrieks and kicking the table as hard as her little legs could pound, flinging herself against me as I held her tightly for the exam. But this was always how she responded to doctors. I learned that day to hold Hannah for what would prove to be a multitude of medical tests.

When Hannah recovered from her illness, she was even further away from us—distant, unsettled, detached. Here she was a year old, and I realized we had completely lost eye contact with her. A few weeks prior, she was beginning to pull herself upright by holding onto our couch. Now, that was gone. I felt a total disconnect from her that I didn't even realize was so pronounced. Her spirit was silent, while her anxiety flared. I would share my concerns at Hannah's fifteen-month checkup, but at the one-year mark, I was still trying to piece it all together or explain it away.

NO BLAME

Even though signs were all around us, we were busy first-time parents and had no idea how truly concerned we should have been. How could we have known? Neither one of us had experience with early childhood—our specialty as educators was with middle school students. We believed Hannah must have been going through a phase or dealing with aftermath from her illness. We were unaware of autism's traits. I don't blame myself or harbor any shame. Nor should you, if you find yourself in the same situation.

Autism awareness is crucial so a parent can get her child the help he or she needs. I hope this theme resonates throughout the book. I want you to do more than notice the differences between your child's behavior and the behavior of kids in the same age range. I want you to know the signs of autism as listed in chapter 1 and pay close attention to developmental milestones. I began to ignore my weekly updates on parenting websites because I believed Hannah was just taking her time. In hindsight, I should have been more suspicious and taken notes on what I observed and thought.

Read through this chapter's text boxes, where you'll find autism screeners for young children both under and over two years of age. If your child manifests any of the behaviors, share concerns with your pediatrician and request a free evaluation from your state's early intervention program. Your pediatrician may also suggest specialists such as developmental pediatricians, child neurologists, and child psychologists or psychiatrists. Always remember, though: even though individuals diagnosed with an autism spectrum disorder (ASD) share a common set of behavioral characteristics, no two individuals will be alike.

Some parents may be in denial—it's understandable, as no one wants to face the possibility of an autism diagnosis. In my case, it wasn't denial. I truly was unaware of the signs. When Hannah's pediatrician suggested autism at her next checkup, I immediately moved forward in getting my daughter the help she so badly needed. Dr. McIntire gave us the precious gift of time.

Whether you're in denial or naïve, act immediately when someone suggests that your child may have autism. The minute you understand that this could be your child's diagnosis, even if it's not official, begin to educate yourself and get help sooner rather than later. Living in denial will make finding the truth so much harder and delay the needed interventions to help your child emerge and grow.

Be gentle with yourself if you're turning the pages of this book and realize you, like me, didn't see the signs or refused to recognize them and take action. Get your child the help he or she needs. Children with autism can't overcome their challenges alone, and delays in identifying and addressing the problem may diminish the effectiveness of treatment and cause them to fall further behind. Autism is notoriously tricky to spot in infants, mainly because the symptoms can mimic other developmental delays. But researchers have come up with some reliable red flags. For example, between six and twelve months, babies who go on to have autism are less likely to smile and vocalize back and forth with parents. They are usually tuned in to things, but not people.

Pride and denial are two emotions that must be put aside to help your child get the professionals they need. I understand pride. We all may think we want our child to be quarterback of the football team, front row hitter in volleyball, valedictorian of the class. However, the child in front of you is one of the best things you've done in all your life. Remember the joy when he or she was born? Focus on helping that child's amazing spirit. As good parents, we want our children to be happy and have the best quality of life. Whether they can voice it or not, our children are counting on us.

"More often than not," says Eustacia Cutler, Temple Grandin's mother, "it is the father's pride that cannot painfully comprehend and fathom such a travesty. 'Tis simply easier to deny or rebuke." Any amount of time a family spends in denial without taking action is time wasted. Their child could be reaping the benefits of early intervention. Get your child help. Maybe you'll discover that your child is only delayed and does not have autism—either way, he or she will be getting useful therapy. I wouldn't want to imagine the remorse a family would face in retrospect at not taking advantage of early intervention. Was it shame? I still know of fathers that won't speak of their child's autism outside of the immediate family.

Those first fifteen months with Hannah mark the era before the worry of a diagnosis. In those first months, we believed our daughter would be able to achieve anything she set her mind to. We were all happy and thought everything was fine. Of course the forty-five-minute commute to my job and my husband's job one hour and fifteen minutes away did wear on us, but our family felt healthy and intact.

Those were days when we could choose what to do instead of being run by therapy schedules and doctors' appointments, when I didn't have to worry about Hannah having a meltdown while working with a doctor or therapist and I wasn't able to comfort her. In those first fifteen months, I could relax when I was tired, instead of having to find a way to continue long after I thought I couldn't. This was the era before I felt I could never do enough.

In those first fifteen months, I didn't feel different and believed my daughter was normal. I liked feeling normal, and I liked thinking my daughter was a normal, typical child. But I'd give up all of that—the freedom to plan my own days, the chance to relax, even that false sense of normal—to have gotten her autism diagnosis sooner. The sooner, the better. That's what I want you to know: the sooner you get your child a diagnosis and the much-needed therapy interventions, the better.

∽ঞ৶৻ **Wisdom from the Round Table** ∽ঞ৶৻

Lori R.: Haircuts used to be just awful for Cameron—the buzzing of the shears caused sheer pain. Even the barber cried, as it broke his heart too. Our occupational therapist then taught us how to help Cameron process the world around him.

Jen: No matter how difficult it was, we never stopped taking Noah outside the house. He disliked shopping because of his sensitivity to noise and would climb under the table in restaurants. A portable DVD player and iPod have been very helpful. Our wherewithal helped Noah overcome his fears. Now, I can proudly say that he is the best shopper ever and even works in a restaurant.

Lori V.: Byron has always been a very literal thinker. In the home, it was very endearing to me; however, people who did not understand Byron did not always find it so. His father once handed him an empty bottle of shampoo and told him to have me put it on our shopping list. He came downstairs, asked where the list was located, and placed the bottle right *on the list.*

Susan: When Tyler was younger he perseverated on anything with wheels, including taking rides in the car. However, he was always so worried about the ride ending that he couldn't enjoy the ride itself.

Karen: John has an **affinity** with all animals, cats especially. It is interesting how autism behaviors correlate with cat behaviors. He would line up shoes, leaving a space in the line for the cat. And you know what? The cat would climb into it. This game would continue with the spot changing and the cat moving into the empty spot.

Sarah: Mitchell is incredibly honest. If I ask him a question, I cherish he will give me an honest answer. I appreciate that in a human being. I can always trust him to follow the rules. Rules give him boundaries.

CHAPTER FOUR

rewriting the script

The Earliest Interventions

A treatment method or an educational method that will work for one child may not work for another child. The one common denominator for all of the young children is that early intervention does work, and it seems to improve prognosis.

—Temple Grandin

March 2007

Today we will get answers for why Hannah has severe food aversions. Her gastroenterologist ordered a swallow/feeding study. This test should show clear evidence as to whether Hannah's food aversions are due to an anatomical problem or oral sensory defensiveness. Mealtimes are more challenging as she ages. On her limited diet, she gags and chokes on food with any substantial texture, and panics with such alarm that she ends up vomiting her entire meal.

My husband and I feel helpless feeding her, which causes arguments and resentment between us. He couldn't come with me today, so my mom came up last night to support us during the procedure.

Unfortunately, on the way to the hospital, Mom missed the exit for the interstate and hasn't answered her cell phone. I don't have time to go back, and she doesn't know how to get to the hospital. Once again, I am alone with Hannah. Hannah's doctor said the test isn't too invasive so we should be fine.

I'm pleased the radiology staff is allowing me to watch the entire procedure. Since I'm at the end of my last trimester, they explain I can watch from behind a glass window with the radiologist. Apparently, the results are going to be immediately visible and conclusive on the screen. I've never before had the convenience of immediate feedback from a radiology test or access to the doctor that reads it.

The speech pathologist is placing Hannah into what looks like a car seat on top of a pole that allows the seat to swivel, like a barber's chair. I should have researched the test's procedure before coming today, but there simply was not time. The radiologist instructs the pathologist to give Hannah a drink of juice. He points out Hannah's swallowing process reflected with her anatomy on the screen. I'm fascinated. Next, the pathologist feeds Hannah yogurt while the radiologist notes the on-screen measurements and Hannah's digestive process.

Hannah is then given a stage-three baby food. I know what's going to happen. I need to get in there to help her. I know this is the reason for the study, but my girl will be absolutely terrified, and I won't be with her. Hannah wants to reject the food, but somehow the pathologist has managed to get it into her mouth. Hannah starts shaking, coughing, and gagging. Her eyes are wide—she's panicking. Then . . . she vomits. I know it's over. She's screaming and wailing.

The radiologist declares that there's nothing anatomically wrong. The issue is her hyper oral defensiveness, but I can't concentrate. I quickly thank him and fling open the door to unbuckle my girl and get us out of here. She dislikes being held, but I can't help it—I hold her tightly in the hallway before allowing her into the stroller, where she's more comfortable, but she's still shivering from fear. I bypass the receptionist on the way out. Not now.

I must find the chapel. Only God can comfort us. The elevator takes us down three floors, Hannah sobbing the entire time, and I see the sign for the chapel up ahead. I open the door and place my back against its petal-shaped louvered glass to roll Hannah's stroller inside the room. I sit on one of the padded chairs and place a hand on Hannah's stroller.

I look at the cross and chalice at the altar, and I pray, pleading. Finally, in the quiet of the space, she is calming, and I'm finally able to cry.

Now I know: nothing's wrong with Hannah's throat structure. Autism is causing her failure to thrive. What more can I do? My little girl needs to grow and develop. How?

For the first time, I feel alone in my search for answers.

The flashback above is an example of the seemingly endless tests Hannah endured during early intervention. We needed answers to help her. I'm comforted by the fact that even with the amazing gift autism gave her memory, she cannot recollect these experiences.

Without a doubt, early intervention helped Hannah. I might go so far as to say early intervention *transformed* Hannah. Early intervention was a great multiplier of impact. An intensive and structured early intervention program focusing on the aspects of language, social pragmatics, behavior, and education was crucial to Hannah's advancements in the years that followed. I refused to sit back and let life happen for Hannah. There was no giving up on her. As Hannah's champion, I strove to set up a process for acquiring skills that would lead to more independence or autonomy. I wasn't fully prepared for what that meant at a practical or logistical level, however. This process turned into almost a full-time job for Hannah and definitely a second full-time job for me. My calendar was out of control! We survived it all, though, and it was worth every sacrifice.

Research agrees that while children are young, their brains are still developing. Their neuropathways can still be shaped. The earlier these pathways are "rewired," the better. Many experts refer to this as "the narrow window of time." Older children have more ingrained behaviors, which makes it more challenging to change habits and tendencies; however, this does not mean the "rewiring" cannot be done even if your child is older than Hannah was when we started intervention. There's no time limit on a person's potential. Development is a lifelong process. Hannah's autism diagnosis was the key that opened the door to understanding.

> ### BENEFITS OF EARLY INTERVENTION[6]
>
> ❋ Provides instruction that builds on your child's strengths to teach new skills, improve behaviors, and remediate areas of weakness.
>
> ❋ Provides information that will help you better understand your child's behavior and needs.
>
> ❋ Offers resources, support, and training that will enable you to work and play with your child more effectively.
>
> ❋ Improves the outcome for your child.

PARENT AS GAME CHANGER

If anyone is going to "rewrite the script" on how autism is going to affect a child, it's the parent. As parents, we are the most influential catalysts in our children's lives. We get the ball rolling on the services our children so desperately need. And there's no time to waste.

In my own right, I became an autism expert. Interventionists become more accountable when parents are educated and prove that they, too, are vested in maximizing results for their children. Knowledge will make you a powerful advocate. Note your child's strengths. Use their passions and interests to stimulate wanted behaviors. An abilities-based model of helping an individual with autism succeed focuses on what the person on the spectrum can do. Concentrating on your child's weaknesses will only produce anxiety and hopelessness in your child. Find out what therapies are available that best serve your child: occupational, physical, speech, developmental, equine-assisted, social/play, feeding, aquatic, music, and behavior management. Think of yourself as a detective in figuring out what your child needs. I felt as if I were unlocking a mystery. The landscape changes so much with available interventions for autism, and we tried an extensive amount as long as they weren't too invasive. Chances are your child won't need as many as Hannah did. Be leery of those so-called professionals that try to "sell" hope. Make sure their programs and interventions are backed by empirical evidence to be worthy of your time, money, and effort. And, most importantly, just because you're feeling overwhelmed and consumed by these demanding activities, don't miss out on *play*. We simply can't go back in time with our children, so let them play—and play with them. Play with them not only when you have a purpose to the play, but also because it's fun for both of you. They may not know how to play. Teach them. They only have one childhood!

As I said in the last chapter and it bears repeating, pride cannot and should not get in the way of our children's early intervention. Our job as parents is to ensure that our children emerge to become the best they can be. So we need to squelch pride to get our kids the help they need. Bad things happen to good people, and that's just how it is. As Professor Randy Pausch, author of *The Last Lecture*, said, "We cannot change the cards we are dealt, just how we play the hand."[7] Pausch was a professor at Carnegie Mellon University. In 2006 he learned he had pancreatic cancer and gave his Last Lecture focusing on what wisdom one would try to impart to the world if it was his or her last chance. His lecture and book stirred a nation. Our children have autism and will always have autism. Our pride will do nothing to help that. The bottom line? Others have been dealt worse hands. Play your hand wisely!

Also, let me remind you that time spent in denial is wasted time during which our children could be getting help. It's tempting to sit too long in denial because you don't want to believe the diagnosis and the unknown is terrifying. Maybe you think it's impossible because autism doesn't run in the family, so you write it off as a phase your child is going through, or you try to convince yourself your child is a "late bloomer." Be honest with yourself. If one specialist has mentioned autism, you're probably going to hear it more and more down the road. Many behaviors associated with autism spectrum disorder aren't behaviors of late bloomers; if you have a typically developing child, you definitely know there is a difference. Autism is not in any family's plan. The behaviors that define our children's autism were out of our control. It's time to come to terms with the diagnosis. Follow my lead.

Do your research. Find what services meet your child's developmental level. Sign them up for the programs and drive them where they need to go. Your Herculean efforts will make a substantial impact on your child. This time next year, they will not be at the same place they are today—thanks to your tireless commitment. When Hannah was two years old, I shared with my grandmother the lost dreams I had for my daughter. Grandma Diefenbach remarked that it was much too early to be writing the end to Hannah's story. I didn't know it at the time, but Grandma was right.

THE EARLIEST THERAPIES: OCCUPATIONAL, PHYSICAL, SPEECH, AND DEVELOPMENTAL

You'll have a lot to figure out in the beginning as you set up all the services and professionals who will be working with your child for weeks, months, or in some cases, years. It feels crazy at first, as you make countless phone calls asking for recommendations and setting up appointments, but it's worth every minute. I promise. Learn more about my process to help you envision your next steps.

FORMING YOUR THERAPY DREAM TEAM

The most effective form of early intervention for Hannah was the in-home therapy she received from First Steps. Although the task was daunting, I didn't allow the paperwork to gather a speck of dust. As soon as Dr. McIntire, our pediatrician, suggested First Steps, I was on the phone, on the computer, talking with the autism consultant in our school district, and reading everything I could get my hands on. Hannah was just a little over fifteen months at this time.

The First Steps evaluation team came out to see if Hannah would qualify. A child with a developmental delay must be at a twenty percent deficit to receive services. The initial evaluators came to our home to evaluate the need for occupational and physical therapy (OT and PT). When they left, they said our caseworker would be calling because they saw a need for Hannah to receive even more services. When the caseworker called to make sure we knew that Hannah qualified for occupational and physical therapy, she said the therapists suggested setting up two more appointments—one to evaluate the need for speech and developmental therapy (ST and DT) and the other for an interview with a children's behavioral psychologist for an official diagnosis of autism. Although our pediatrician had suspected autism and Hannah had an upcoming visit with a neurologist, First Steps was offering an official diagnosis.

I was numb. I opened my calendar, thought about my schedule, tried to absorb the fact that they, too, saw the autism, and received directions to choose our therapists for the services Hannah had already qualified for: OT and PT. I felt an overwhelming panic lurch inside, but I had no time for it. The woman on the phone seemed kind and this call was extremely important, but didn't she know what she had just unloaded on me? In two weeks I had gone from being a naïve mom to a master scheduler, and soon I'd be a therapy aficionado, as Hannah would go on to also qualify for ST and DT.

My husband and I realized we needed to move closer to our jobs. I couldn't teach and make it home in time for Hannah to receive services when the latest therapy appointment for the day was at 5:00. With the commute, Hannah and I rarely made it home before 5:15.

We put our home up for sale—the home in which we had planned to raise our family. It sold in three days. We had to pack up and move at the same time the fall semester of school was ready to begin. We were also planning for the arrival of our son in March. Although genetic counseling and testing didn't have the ability to determine autism, we wanted to make sure we were prepared for any other identifiable challenges if he had them. All prenatal tests came back typical.

I sought out the best therapists for Hannah, but what did I know about therapy? I compared therapist against therapist based on their experience, philosophy, and expertise, and identified those that looked strongest. But some therapists that looked great on paper already had full caseloads or only worked during the day. As a mother who worked outside of the home, I felt jilted. In some instances, I called my preferred therapists anyway and pleaded Hannah's case. I knew it wouldn't hurt. After a lot of calls, some of them made exceptions, and I finally put together Hannah's "Therapy Dream Team." It was time for the therapy merry-go-round.

Each therapist that would come to our home would give me a small list of actions to take within that next week. I watched what the therapists did, and then I modeled it for Hannah. As a teacher, I felt like not doing my "homework" would truly let my daughter down, and I wouldn't see the gains I was hoping to see. That would be on me. So I created daily task lists and repeated skills that Hannah had mastered because if we didn't, she would lose them. We worked hard to meet the high expectations of our therapists who had agreed to meet with Hannah during their off hours or when their caseloads were already full. We no longer had privacy in our home. Our front door was a revolving door for Hannah's therapists. We had zero flexibility in our weekly schedule, but I would soon learn that routine was a requirement that best served Hannah's needs anyway. Spontaneity was a thing of the past. We adjusted our life to the parameters of ASD.

COMMUNICATION WITH PROVIDERS

* Discuss with each therapist the goals of the other therapists and information provided by doctors.
* Make sure daycare is on board with the dietary and/or sensory modulation plan.
* All interventionists and daycare providers should be aware of prescribed medication.
* A communication log should travel back and forth between daycare and home. This maximizes efficiency and allows the provider and parent to exchange pertinent, daily information.
* Be as specific as possible about any of your child's troubling behaviors so interventionists can provide guidance.
* Don't be afraid to question your providers and take notes.

OCCUPATIONAL THERAPY

Tara, Hannah's occupational therapist, was committed to Hannah and our family—and just as stubborn as Hannah. Every therapist uses tools and approaches appropriate for a particular child's struggles. Tara's methods, patience, and wisdom in discerning what Hannah needed at each stage amazed me. She had a vehicle full of therapy tools, selecting what she felt would help Hannah progress to the next goal. Sometimes Tara and I would take two trips out to her car to gather all of her materials and equipment for each session.

Right away Tara recognized Hannah's sensory processing disorder. Food textures, auditory stimuli, skin sensitivity, **oral sensory dysfunction**, proprioception issues, **vestibular** challenges, and motor planning all gave Hannah problems. I would have never known this so soon if it weren't for Tara. She gave me the book *The Out-of-Sync Child* and told me she would be giving me many more resources that were optional to read, but this one was mandatory. The book described Hannah perfectly, providing the explanation for why my daughter never wanted me to touch her or even hold her as a baby. Sock seams would always drive Hannah crazy. When she found her voice around three and a half, she would just cry and say, "Ooey, ooey." The change of seasons into warmer clothes bothered her. Going from short sleeves to long sleeves and shorts to long pants was excruciating to her. I still remember her face when the long sleeves would touch her skin: Pain—an overwhelming flood of sensation. I can't imagine an existence where everything you see, hear, and feel is magnified to a painful intensity.

As soon as Tara arrived she would start sessions using sensory modulation, swinging Hannah on the playset in the back yard (even in cold weather). Other times she would wrap Hannah up in a blanket, and then the two of us would swing her, perform joint compressions, or implement the Wilbarger Brushing Protocol (brushing the body with a small surgical brush throughout the day) to decrease Hannah's sensory defensiveness. This was all part of Hannah's **sensory diet**. Tara introduced a huge Rubbermaid tub full of rice, but it was sensory overload for Hannah, so we had to start with something larger: navy beans. In the beginning, Hannah was scared to touch, scoop, and shovel them. Tara would hide small objects such as toy animals that Hannah adored, and Hannah would cry painfully just removing the beans from covering the animals. Once Hannah's receptors adjusted and Tara was able to actually place Hannah in the Rubbermaid container with the beans, Hannah graduated to the rice. And we had to start all over.

Hannah's worst fear was to touch or be touched by something wet or something with the consistency of yogurt or applesauce—if that happened, she would scream, cry, flap, and look at it as if it were a hot coal burning right through her skin. These issues were part of the reason she didn't want to eat. Tara started with having Hannah touch soap bubbles on our kitchen table. Like so many things, Hannah found this painful. Little by little over the next two years, Hannah was able to spread the bubbles over the table and eventually touch Jell-O and yogurt.

Hannah's oral sensory dysfunction presented many problems. It was a battle to get a toothbrush into her mouth. In fact, she wouldn't let anything into her mouth. With proprioceptive problems, Hannah had no idea where her body was in space, so here she was between two and three years old and still had not put anything into her mouth herself, not with a spoon nor with her hands. To address this, Tara used many techniques to desensitize Hannah's receptors, strengthen her mouth for chewing, and organize her body to acknowledge its position.

Tara used what's called a chewy tube that gave Hannah an oral motor workout. At first Hannah resisted having it in her mouth, but she slowly accepted it. Tara also made sure Hannah had access to a Tripp Trapp chair that would put Hannah in the best position to eat and it would make her feel as though she was supported in all areas of her body.

When Hannah started talking, around three and a half years old, Tara would have her count Cheerios; place pretzel sticks to her head acting as bull's horns and "moo"; bring a Dum Dum sucker to her mouth to kiss; and play with shaving cream, whipped cream, and finger paint. All of these activities helped Hannah at least get food closer to her lips. She would later learn to hold a spoon. At first she worked on feeding a doll baby, then Tara used **video modeling** to help Hannah learn to scoop her oatmeal. However, because of her proprioception struggles, Hannah struggled to bring the spoon straight to her mouth. A heavy spoon solved the problem. We found video modeling was the only way at this age for Hannah to learn from others. Any other time, she was in her own world and paid no attention to what others were doing. Tara also used personalized, short stories she had created to help Hannah understand the importance of several life skills like tooth brushing. Carol Gray, author and consultant to children, adolescents, and adults with autism, developed something similar, Social Stories, in 1990. They are used as a tool to help individuals on the autism spectrum better understand the nuances of interpersonal communication so that they can interact in an effective and appropriate manner.

Sensory and mouth strength profiles gave Tara data to see numerically how Hannah was improving. Though Hannah was learning the physical movements to eat, she needed to take in more calories. Every morsel that went into her mouth either our daycare provider or I had to almost force in. She would vomit practically every day, most often after dinner—the heaviest meal. When discussing this with others not familiar with our situation, they would say, "She'll eat when she's hungry." Instead of correcting, I would pretend to agree. It was easier than disagreeing: "Well, no, she really won't. If you'd like to try that method out, we'll just watch my daughter starve to death."

In addition to Tara's in-home therapy, when Connor was a baby and Hannah was two years old, we also started seeing the Feeding Team at Riley Children's Hospital once a week on Mondays—right after I got off work, and before her developmental therapy in the evening.

Getting there involved picking up the kids at the sitter, commuting thirty-five minutes to the hospital, unloading the stroller and loading in Connor, navigating the two kids through the tight parking garage and safely onto the elevator—all while struggling with Hannah, who disliked touch and, after she had learned to walk, pulled her hand from mine and wandered constantly. She obsessively pressed the elevator button, but refused to get on when the doors opened for fear of stepping on a line, which, in Hannah's world, was not allowed. She despised the hospital's automatic doors and would try to run from them. In fact, she would run from me often, unafraid of strangers, so I always had to be vigilant not to lose her. By the time we avoided all the lines and automatic doors throughout the hospital, I was mentally and physically exhausted. Yet at that same time, Connor would be ready to bust out of the stroller. We endured this process once a week for two years.

At feeding therapy, staff would monitor Hannah's weekly food intake and nutrition, work on eating with Hannah, and give me pointers that helped her gradually improve. One of the most important fortunes of our time there, however, was what her feeding therapist told me. She was the first person to tell me she felt Hannah had a higher aptitude or intellectual ability than her neurologist believed. She was the first autism expert to express the possibility that Hannah could experience significant advances. I had never heard this before.

Hope.

Hannah also had a lot of trouble with crossing **midline**, an imaginary line separating the sides of the body. She struggled with motor planning (the ability to conceive, plan, and carry out an act) and upper body strength, making it a challenge to do certain things like hook her own seatbelt, open doors, give herself a bath, and get dressed. I never knew the huge role crossing midline played in a child's development. Tara broke down the motor planning process of putting on a shirt into nine steps: Lay shirt on floor. Back faces you. Tag on top. Separate bottom of shirt. Pull over head. Hold left bottom of shirt with right hand. Place left hand into shirt and through left arm hole. Hold right bottom of shirt with left hand. Place right hand into shirt and through the left arm hole. Hannah memorized each step and practiced with Tara, then reviewed it each morning with me. Only when Connor reached a similar age did I realize typical kids find the process of dressing a natural, easy process. Unbelievable.

When Hannah was three years old, long after our state's therapy expired, we hired Tara to stay as Hannah's private occupational therapist once a week for an hour. We scraped to afford the extra services because she was so valuable to Hannah's treatment. Tara continued to help us with eating, tooth brushing, toilet training, and bathing, so Hannah could build skills to function with increasing independence.

PHYSICAL THERAPY

A lot of kids begin walking with their parents at a very young age—the adult holds the child's hands above their head. When we tried that with Hannah, she would go limp, like she didn't even know there was a floor beneath her. At Gymboree, I had watched countless kids go through the stage of pulling themselves up and beginning to walk, passing Hannah. The actual act of pulling up was symbolized as First Steps' logo. How is it that that one simple symbol could evoke such emotional distress for me? Hannah would just continue to army crawl with little interest in pulling up, especially after an upper respiratory infection at fourteen months. I began to wonder if she would ever walk. Gross motor difficulties are usually not associated with autism; however, in retrospect, I believe this served as a "red flag" to our pediatrician that something was wrong with our daughter.

According to Hannah's physical therapist, Jennifer, Hannah had several problems that were causing her not to walk. The first and most important was that Hannah had a proprioception problem—she really had no idea where her body was in space. Jennifer said that Hannah could not feel the ground under her feet, and if she couldn't feel the floor, of course she wouldn't want to walk. Jennifer had therapies to help and predicted Hannah, who was seventeen months at the time, would walk within a year.

Jennifer would physically stand behind Hannah and put her hands around Hannah's underarms. She would then lean Hannah back on her and drag her feet across the floor to help her recognize the sensation of a floor below. Jennifer also recommended new orthotics available on trial called Suresteps. Used mostly on children with Down syndrome, the orthotics would be tailored for Hannah's feet and provide the sensory input that her feet needed. I'd Velcro them together at the top of the foot over Hannah's socks, then place her shoes over them. Two months after wearing the Suresteps, Hannah pulled up on a child's play shopping cart. She then proceeded to take a few steps. A few steps turned into methodical laps that started in the kitchen, proceeded into the dining room, picked up speed in the entryway, and confidently made her way back to the kitchen—only to start all over again without looking up.

Hannah also needed to improve her leg strength. Doing laps around the house with the grocery cart would provide some strength conditioning, but Jennifer supplemented by having Hannah do step-ups on a small kid's stool and stand up from a child-sized chair while Jennifer held her hand for balance.

Hannah needed to improve her motor planning and vestibular sense, or balance, so Jennifer would position her to pull up on the ottoman, moving the beloved grocery cart so that if Hannah pulled up on the ottoman, all she had to do was reach for the cart. Jennifer would not allow her to crawl over to it. After helping Hannah for three months with the steps to pulling up, Hannah got it just before her second birthday.

Yes, Hannah learned to walk—on carpet. Unfortunately, when she tried to transfer onto the kitchen tile floor from the family room's Berber carpet, she fell. We worked on learning that transition. Then there was the yard. Jennifer explained that outside, the grass was so uneven compared to carpet or tile, Hannah sensed she was always stepping into a deep hole like a roller coaster sensation. Once Hannah mastered walking in the grass, she struggled to transition from the grass to the flat-surfaced patio. That confused me because the patio should've been a welcome relief after the uneven yard.

Eventually, she walked over every surface. In fact, Hannah got so comfortable and confident that, as I described her behavior at Riley Hospital when we went in for food therapy, she became a "runner" and would just take off in public places. Individuals with autism never feel at ease about where they are—so they run away in search of a location where they feel at ease. Hannah had no inherent feeling of the security of staying with me. I'm certain that if lost, she would have been unaffected and unafraid, which terrified us. Through a service provided by Riley Children's Hospital, we obtained several items, including a GPS device that Hannah wore on her wrist and a tracker for the adult who was with her. If Hannah did get away from us, she could be found. In addition, we purchased the "Mommy I'm Here Child Alert Locator," which attached to her shoelaces. This was only used if we knew there was no possibility she would be more than 150 feet away. All we had to do was press an alert button, and her shoe would start beeping very loudly. In addition to these high-tech gadgets, we added a low-tech solution: a small, laminated card safety-pinned to her shirt with her name, diagnosis, and our cell numbers.

Next-level physical therapy aggravated Hannah. Her motor planning was too slow to kick and catch a ball—her mind couldn't plan fast enough for her feet and hands to kick or clasp the ball. It would roll past and she'd scream in frustration. She couldn't jump well either because of limited muscle strength.

Hannah's therapist met us at the park to help her use the playground equipment. A fun outing, Hannah improved her motor planning, built confidence and strength, and enjoyed the experience of just being a kid. I, too, enjoyed watching her at the playground. For a few minutes, I was a regular mom at the playground with her children—except Hannah still had to learn even simple things like how to sit at the top of a slide and position herself to go down. But I loved watching her. For other moms, it seemed so basic. For me, it made her seem "just like one of the kids."

SPEECH THERAPY

Our speech therapist, Laquita, took a dynamic approach to wooing Hannah into our world. Her exaggerated facial expressions, intonation of voice, and knowledge of **floortime** and **applied behavior analysis (ABA)** therapies exposed Hannah to best practices while taking a conservative and more realistic approach at times, using only tools like the **Picture Exchange Communication System (PECS)**. Since Hannah could not communicate with words, she could express her needs and make choices using these cards. I would place two cards in front of Hannah and say "I want," and then she would choose one of the cards. Until Hannah was five years old, we used these PECS cards and sign language to communicate. This ensured that Hannah felt some degree of independence and pride.

Even though Hannah stayed silent until about three and a half years of age, we could see she was fascinated with animals (especially cats and cows), classical music from her Baby Einstein DVDs (music served as an organized focus—like a carrier signal), numbers, shapes, colors, astronomy, and books. She adored flash cards, so to try to generate language, I showed her cards over and over again depicting the themes that most interested her. At three and a half, she began to produce words based on those cards, using her gift of memorization. I read to her constantly. Our favorite book was *You Are My I Love You*. After every two lines I would always leave out the last word, which rhymed with the previous line, and she began to speak it. This book formed an important part of her bedtime ritual and led to her saying the most wonderful three words ever: I love you! These were words that at one time I wasn't sure I would ever hear. Seeing the power of memorization and reading, I followed the same process with popular books like *The Very Hungry Caterpillar* and *Goodnight Moon*. Soon she could say "egg," "pop," "plums," as well as "bears," "chairs," "kittens," and "mittens." And "balloon" and "moon."

I would count for Hannah in the car and sing "Old MacDonald." Before long she would make animal sounds and count! I kept encouraging her to count higher just to hear her voice. She could count to two hundred well before she could put two words spontaneously together. Numbers were predicatable for Hannah because they never changed. One day while pushing the kids through our neighborhood in the double stroller, I heard Hannah randomly saying numbers. I celebrated when I discovered she was reading the house numbers on the mailboxes. What must have seemed like minor progress to others—or nothing more than memorization—we celebrated as victories. Hearing her voice, even for small moments, continued to give me hope.

Laquita moved to Ohio. The therapist who replaced her only brought two board games. Nothing else. You really don't know how great a therapist is until you get a bad one. In her notes the replacement therapist described Hannah as non-engaged, unmotivated, fussy, and lazy. But the therapist didn't do a thing to make even the two board games exciting and went on to talk about how smart and outgoing her son was—who happened to be the same age as Hannah. If there were more speech therapists available, I would've made a change; unfortunately, this wasn't the case. Don't be afraid to make a switch if the setting isn't conducive for your child. Early intervention is a very vulnerable age for children.

I'd hear the incessant chatter of other kids Hannah's age and was stunned that it was so easy for them. Why did Hannah have so much trouble producing and understanding language? Why couldn't she just open her mouth and speak her thoughts like the others? Comparison stole my joy. It seemed unfair she had to work so hard, but we kept at it. I believed she would one day be able to speak freely. Others shared their doubts, but I didn't let them drag me down. Hannah would find her voice; we would find it together.

DEVELOPMENTAL THERAPY

We had to fit in developmental therapy with Lisa once a week for an hour, just like Hannah's OT, PT, ST, and feeding therapy. Through developmental therapy, we hoped to see Hannah achieve eye contact, engage in playing with toys using joint attention, learn functional daily skills, and increase imaginative play. Basically, therapy would guide her brain to motor plan in an entirely different way than it naturally behaved, releasing Hannah from the ever-present anxiety that haunted her.

Even at age two and a half, Hannah hadn't developed the fine motor skills or strength needed to put together Mr. Potato Head, string large beads on a rope, flip or turn a switch to get an animal to pop up on a popular toddler toy, place oversized golf tees into holes, or coordinate mouth muscles, lips, and breath to blow bubbles. So she practiced these activities, session after session. The therapist recommended we make a simple toy: My dad drilled a hole in the lid of a peanut butter jar so Hannah could stuff pompoms of various sizes through the opening, which helped her proprioception and gave her practice with her pincer grasp. In time, she could string the beads, position the golf tees, and even work large jigsaw puzzles. Clipping clothespins to a piece of cardboard built strength and coordination that helped her master Mr. Potato Head and turn the switch on pop-up toys. Hannah became frustrated when working with the bubbles, so we had her try to master blowing feathers off of a book first. That took continual practice. Like everything else, Hannah had to work harder at it than other kids her age.

WAYS TO MAKE A DIFFERENCE FOR YOUR CHILD
- ❖ Become the expert on autism.
- ❖ Talk to other parents that have children on the spectrum.

- Find out what services are available in your area.
- Find out what services are *not* available in your area.
- There is strength in numbers. Find out about the Autism Society of America and Autism Speaks and consider joining one that feels like the best fit for you.
- Become a partner in your child's education.
- Get involved with your providers.
- Keep records organized in an accordion folder.
- Ask for help from friends/family.
- Begin to think ahead to your child's further education, employment, and later life challenges.

ADDITIONAL THERAPY, DOCTORS, AND TESTS

The previous therapies were foundational, but they aren't the only options. We found other therapies to help Hannah emerge and turned to even more doctors and tests. As you'll see, we explored every possibility to create the best possible outcome for our daughter. I hope it gives you ideas of the kinds of help your child can get.

SOCIAL/PLAY THERAPY

Hannah participated in social/play therapy offered in six-week intervals every summer until she turned five. A licensed occupational therapist ran the program through a social services company in our county. Play was an excellent vehicle to provide exposure to social interactions. Children's experiences and knowledge are often communicated through play. Even if I didn't see marked improvement at the time, the experience would later prove to be beneficial.

A TRIP TO THE AUDIOLOGIST

We took Hannah to an audiologist for a hearing test. How would a hearing test be performed on a child who was unable to talk? The audiologist led us to an audiology chamber, where I was positioned on a stool and Hannah had to sit on my lap. We were surrounded by a monkey with cymbals, a bird that flapped its wings and chirped, and were bombarded by sounds from the left and right with different tones and volumes. Hannah's ability to look in the direction of each sound was the actual test. She passed this test with no problem. Although we found one area where she didn't have to struggle, in hindsight I realized First Steps was actually ruling out a hearing problem as the cause for her delays. I could only wish that Hannah's challenges could be fixed by a set of ear tubes.

DEVELOPMENTAL PEDIATRICIAN, GASTROENTEROLOGIST, AND DIETITIAN

Because of Hannah's walking and eating delays, the neurologist sent us to a developmental pediatrician who wanted to do an MRI of Hannah's spine and brain to rule out seizure activity, loss of white matter, and oxygen deprivation at birth. The doctor was also concerned about her reflexes and a dimple at the bottom of her spine. Once again, I was alone at this meeting and all of these words sounded ominous. My quest for answers led to more questions. Another appointment for the MRI needed to be made, insurance to be processed, and another day of work to be missed. And, unfortunately, Hannah would have to be sedated. The MRI scan conclusively proved there was no physical evidence of any other medical anomalies for Hannah. What a relief!

The developmental pediatrician thought we should also see a gastroenterologist and dietitian due to Hannah's eating challenges and digestion problems—she strained while going to the bathroom and her tummy was distended. Her system had slowed down to a standstill and her pediatrician had already prescribed two enemas be done at home—awful and traumatic. I know this procedure isn't just done on kids with autism, but no parent should have to perform that unnatural and violating procedure. It made sense that she wouldn't want to eat if food was not going through her system. More appointments and phone calls.

The gastroenterologist disproved structural throat abnormalities with the swallow/feeding study, and the dietitian made a few suggestions for calorie intake like supplementing with Carnation Instant Breakfast and mentioned an over-the-counter medicine that would help her digest food properly. She reassured me that I was doing the best I could to get food into my little girl—for one moment, I felt understood and affirmed by her compassionate words. And, once again, I hugged a complete stranger who told me I wasn't doing a thing wrong.

BEHAVIORAL PSYCHOLOGIST

Hannah and I continued to see the behavioral psychologist from First Steps that diagnosed her autism. She offered strategies for arranging situations to cause less confusion for Hannah's motor planning. We hoped this would reduce the frequency of Hannah's meltdowns—the number of outbursts was increasing as a result of all the uncomfortable therapies and sensory difficulties. I needed strategies to avoid the outbursts, control her during them when they couldn't be avoided, and discuss them with her afterward.

Some of the sessions focused on what I had to change, and less about what Hannah had to change. The psychologist wanted us to create a steady atmosphere for Hannah, so I suddenly had to redirect rituals I had done the same way for thirty-seven years—like how we now needed a visual schedule of the morning routine that did not allow for flexibility, and I needed to simplify language in a way that made it more meaningful to Hannah—fewer words using only the subject and the verb. She also suggested a gluten-free, casein-free diet and the addition of fish oil. Because Hannah already had a limited diet, this was not an option. I questioned whether or not a controlled environment was possible for Hannah in the future. The psychologist reminded me Hannah was not even three years old, so we should create this space now, at this young age; she assured me there was plenty of time for Hannah to overcome a lot of her anxiety-causing triggers in the future. Through interactions with Hannah's behavioral therapist, I learned to extend grace to all parents that have an child that is out of sync with their surroundings—it's not necessarily noncompliance.

COPING STRATEGIES FOR PARENTS AS CAREGIVERS

* Join an autism support group. They understand.
* Don't forget to take care of yourself—exercise, sleep, treat yourself to a massage and manicure.
* Journal your feelings and fears.
* Don't allow yourself to obsess about what caused the autism. As of this writing, no one knows the cause, so you're wasting precious energy.
* Seek professional advice from a counselor.
* Allow your child to be "autistic."
* Not everyone needs to know your child's label.
* Take a vacation without your child who has autism.
* Cherish your marriage.
* Online forums can be a source of strength for many reasons.

THE PARENT'S STRUGGLE

We worked hard to see Hannah make many small steps during this first stage of intervention, from fifteen months to age three. I learned to celebrate the smallest successes, because she did make progress even when it was minuscule. We celebrated *inchstones* instead of milestones. I believe that's the reason compliments come easy for special needs parents. We notice small accomplishments in big ways. Would the second stage of Hannah's intervention, from age three to six, bring continued growth in my girl?

One time Dr. Pappas, our neurologist, wasn't able to see us at our appointment, so his assistant stepped in. Her first question was the same as my husband's father, "How do you feel about Hannah being on the autism spectrum?" I stared at her. I'm a special needs parent. Would a medical professional actually ask me that? How did she think I felt about Hannah being on the spectrum? I felt sad, cheated, angry, and jealous of other parents. Is that what she wanted to hear? Maybe I should have told her I wake up in the middle of the night painfully reminded that my daughter will probably not walk down the aisle or attend my college alma mater. I just looked at my husband and said, "Do not put me through this." After the assistant left to get the doctor, she returned with yet another informative packet on autism, as if I didn't have enough.

Special needs parents need to be listened to without feeling judged. They sometimes need to vent. Sometimes we're close to a meltdown ourselves. A couple of times I even had the audacity to correct others' mistakes and let them know how I felt in a not-so-nice way. In retrospect, that was wrong of me. My life was strenuous enough without others causing more discontentment. Special needs parents need to be understood when they say they're physically and emotionally exhausted. They need a time out. Day after day, I felt completely drained. I had to get more comfortable with having less control. Sometimes when I cried, no one saw my tears. However, I knew I had to keep going. I had a well-worn social armor. Saying I was fine never meant I was fine. I had to wake up the next day and do more things, lots of things, so I would need to find the strength. Autism is not for the weak-hearted.

We have to believe that our children will improve. They will improve because we will get them all the doctors, therapists, and social play groups that will help with whatever they need. That's what keeps us going. Our efforts will bring progress. You'll see.

When Hannah was first diagnosed with autism, our school system's psychologist, with a son on the spectrum, paid me a visit. Upon walking into my classroom, she handed me a poem entitled "Welcome to Holland" by Emily Pearl Kingsley. If you haven't read it, you should. The poem compares having a child with special needs to the experience of getting on an airplane for a trip. You believe you're headed for Venice, but then the stewardess tells you that you've landed in Holland. Well, you can spend your time crying for the gondolas, streamers, masks, and Venetian glass, or you can get out and enjoy all the tulips and windmills. It's not quite what you had expected, but it is lovely just the same—an excellent metaphor.

∾⧢ᴥ **Wisdom from the Round Table** ∾⧢ᴥ

Lori R.: There has been a team of experts to help Cameron overcome many obstacles, and I believe God placed them into our lives.

Jen: Speech therapy gave Noah a voice—communication with his peers and reading skills improved. Occupational therapy was also integral—as it helped Noah with fine motor skills, writing, and decreased his sensory defensiveness.

Lori V.: Support mechanisms for parents are critical. Parents may not believe there's time, but in order to take care of our children, we must also take care of ourselves.

Susan: Our family made the choice not to do therapy all five days a week. Tyler may have more skills if we had. However, with my role as a wife and a mother to another child, I did not think this was best for our situation. I believe this decision helped our family remain strong and intact.

Karen: No matter where a child lies on the spectrum, all forms of autism have disruptive behaviors and time-consuming treatments.

Sarah: Since most of Mitchell's struggles, social and organizational, presented later in life, he hasn't had much in the area of therapy. It has been important for us to push Mitchell to try things that are hard, while still providing support in the background. For example, this year he has joined the marching band. Through this experience, he is learning that hard work, dedication, and perseverance can pay off. To support him in the background, we've had to give him space when he's home, lessen his workload in other areas, and just allow him to vent when he needs to. He is growing tremendously.

CHAPTER FIVE

a baby boy is born

Sibling Relationships

Siblings are the longest relationship you'll have in your life.
They know the good times, the bad, the neuroses, all that shared
history.

—Tiffany Shlain

March 2007
Yesterday at 12:06 p.m., Connor Matthew made his way into the world.
His cry, his curly, strawberry-blond hair, his strong upper body, his
flailing long arms and legs, and his blue eyes all told me he was going
to be okay—nothing to worry about. The peace I felt in that delivery
room was a gift. Thank you, Connor.

Several family members and friends popped into our hospital room
to meet and hold Connor. Visitors brought balloon bouquets and flow-
ers, and we asked them to sign a picture mat and add words of well
wishes just as we'd arranged at his sister's birth. Every few hours my
husband entertained our visitors in the hallway while I nursed our
baby boy.

This morning, the day after Connor's delivery, I awake early be-
cause our pediatrician, Dr. McIntire, said he would be on the north side
of town first thing. He wasn't kidding. He's here at 7:00 to do Connor's

examination. He assures me all of Connor's newborn screenings and hearing tests are fine, and he'll be released to go home tomorrow.

Around 10:00, my obstetrician, Dr. Gaudreau, comes in to check on me. She coos over Connor and marvels that I've already dressed him in a blue-striped, long-sleeved, buttoned-up Gap onesie with matching cap and socks. I point to the stuffed basketball, football, and baseball in the hospital bassinet. "Lori, once again, you have all of your bases covered." We all laugh at the intended pun. Then her face softens, and she offers that same caring look she gave me eight months ago when we first met.

Eight months ago, I walked into her office as a new patient because my obstetrician had retired. While waiting for the appointment, I'd worked myself into a tizzy so that by the time she walked in, I blurted out, "My husband and I have a daughter. We wanted to have another child. I've always wanted a boy. We thought it would take some time because we had fertility problems with our daughter, but it didn't. I'm pregnant. Last month our sixteen-month-old daughter got a preliminary diagnosis of autism. I'm devastated. We're so happy about this pregnancy, but scared at the same time. Can you help me?" Her calm, reassuring, and informative presence has given me strength from that moment on.

As I hand Connor off to my husband, I realize something. I've been holding him since his feeding at 8:30 and he hasn't fussed, wiggled in his blanket, or cried. Not once! His tiny little lips even have a pursed grin on them, and he's looking me in the eyes! He is looking me in the eyes!

After examining me, Dr. Gaudreau agrees we're good to leave tomorrow and congratulates us one last time. We thank her for her kindness. Although there are no genetic tests for autism, during my pregnancy, we wanted to be aware of any potential challenges our baby may encounter; therefore, Dr. Gaudreau agreed to genetic counseling and in utero testing for our baby. All of our counseling and testing proved clear for any problems. I'm not certain other doctors would have been kind enough to do the same.

After lunch at 1:00, my husband and I anxiously await Hannah's arrival with my mom. Mom has been watching Hannah since early

*yesterday morning, so I'll bet Hannah misses us. I know we miss her!
She's going to meet her new baby brother, Connor! I hope she's care-
ful around him. She loves books, so I've bought and wrapped* I'm a Big
Sister *for her. Two-year-old Hannah has just learned to walk with her
Surestep orthotics. She's a little wobbly, but I hope Mom has her walk
into the hospital room. What a big moment this is going to be!*

*At 1:30 we hear Mom talking to Hannah outside of the room, and
we both smile. There's a knock on the door. "Come in!" I yell, hoping
she'll recognize my voice. Connor is swaddled in a blanket in my arms,
and my husband is standing right beside our bed. The door opens, and
here she comes. Her long hair is gathered at the top of her head in a large
pink bow. She's wearing a white T-shirt that has a little girl on the front
wearing a polka-dotted dress, with Hannah's hair color and a bow. The
shirt reads, "I'm the Big Sister." How fun! Mom must have bought that
for her. Hannah's wearing blue jeans and her K-Swiss tennis shoes.*

*Her gait is steady—intentional—and her eyes are wide. I call her
name. "Hannah!" She looks at the knobs on the bed, which are at her
height. She touches them. She turns and walks away from the bed—
then begins flapping her arms and hands. She turns again and walks
toward the couch and looks at the balloons and flowers and out the
window. I say her name, but louder: "Hannah! Come see your new
baby brother, Connor."*

*Nothing. We have not seen her in a day and a half, and there's no
response to either of our voices or our faces. My husband, hoping to
console me, sweeps Hannah up from behind and places her on the bed.
Instead of looking at either of us, she finds the food stand on the other
side of the bed, crawls over my legs, places a hand on it, and is upset
when it rolls away.*

*I sob. Why did I bother imagining this would play out any differ-
ently? Why doesn't she even acknowledge her own mother and father,
and her new little brother? She's a big sister! Doesn't she even realize
that?*

Of course she doesn't.

*And I wail so loudly that within minutes, the hospital chaplain
walks into our room—no doubt summoned by the nurses' station near
my room. Exhausted by these postpartum sobs, I realize that even when*

blessed with the miracle of life, I can be reduced to tears. I feel pain or grief so sharp and deep, I cry until the hurt is numbed.

As the tears subside, the chaplain says a prayer and excuses himself. I look over, and Hannah is now on the couch holding her present. I carefully get out of bed, take Connor with me, and decide to help her unwrap her book. We join her in her world in hopes of bringing her into our family's new world of four.

There is no doubt that siblings raised with a brother or sister with autism spectrum disorder (ASD) are influenced by significant, unique, and challenging experiences. Over time, Hannah started to show an interest in her brother and not an outright disregard of him. I would have to be satisfied. The scene above was just the beginning for us. Connor only knows life with his sister's autism, where adjustments to plans are always possible.

Parents often underestimate autism's effect on typical siblings. After the incident at Connor's birth, I resolved to manage my expectations for all future exchanges between my two kids: Whatever tone or atmosphere my daughter sets in a room, I would not allow it to affect my relationship with my son. And that started my core conviction that Connor's childhood wouldn't be overshadowed by his sister's needs. Don't allow your typical children to be pushed into the background, either! They deserve to be nurtured, loved, and valued. I would never want my son's contempt. His love is too important to me for him to harbor bitter feelings.

It's hard. We can only do so much with the resources we have. As moms, we tend to think everything is our fault anyway, but it's not—we're only human. The helpful hints are to serve only as reminders, as they are impossible to follow all of the time and in all circumstances. Typical siblings will no doubt be both strengthened and stressed by having a brother or sister on the spectrum. Age, temperament, personality, birth order, gender, parental attitudes, and supports all play a role in autism's effect on the typical sibling—not to mention the level of functioning of the sibling with autism. My experience has been with the middle to upper level of the spectrum; however, the practical guidelines suggested in this chapter are valuable for every level of the spectrum but with discernible efficacy. In her memoir, *Ketchup is My Favorite Vegetable: A Family Grows Up With Autism*, Liane Kupferberg Carter states, "Siblings are the profoundly unsung heroes of autism. They are the children who grow up in therapists' waiting rooms, learning lessons in self-sacrifice far too soon."

A FAMILY OF FOUR

We were happy when we discovered we were expecting our second child; however, we were also troubled because the pregnancy coincided with beginning the path to Hannah's autism diagnosis. At thirty-six, my biological clock was ticking. We liked the idea of our children being two years apart. We never imagined we would conceive so quickly and easily, but that's always been the journey with Connor—nothing but easy.

Hannah's neurologist, Dr. Pappas, was able to ease our minds on the chances of our second child also having autism. Dr. Gaudreau also soothed our worry by allowing us genetic counseling and in utero testing. The most moving information from the testing was that we were going to have a little boy. As you may recall from earlier, I'd always wanted a boy. Despite the odds Dr. Pappas provided, I was frightened because at this point I knew the chances of our child having autism increased significantly—boys are four times more likely to have autism than girls. The worry was there throughout the months leading up to Connor's birth, but I tried to keep it at bay. I actually had no choice. With teaching full-time, Hannah's therapies and doctors' appointments, and our recent move, my time and mind—even my emotions—were tapped out. I forced myself to focus only on the positive of my pregnancy.

Once again, we had a wonderful time decorating the nursery and preparing for our son's arrival. We had a friend come over and paint his walls with a sports theme: a crimson Indiana University football helmet, a baseball jersey with our last name across the back, and a basketball swishing through a net. I selected sports-related books for his bookshelf: one about Peyton Manning, Michael Jordan, and Alex

Rodriguez. A baseball nightlight, a basketball beanbag, and a sports-themed growth chart made great accents.

In March, I took off the week prior to Connor being induced, but instead of relaxing and anticipating his birth, I spent the entire week researching autism and took Hannah for her swallow/feeding study.

Cindy was assigned as my labor and delivery nurse again—the same nurse who helped deliver Hannah. The Pitocin worked much faster this time, and I was allowed my epidural four hours sooner than with Hannah. I remember Cindy paged Dr. Gaudreau to say that I was ready. Dr. Gaudreau came in and said she would change into her scrubs and then we'd deliver this baby. Cindy said, "There is no time to get into your scrubs. This baby is coming now!"

MILESTONES REACHED

Connor hit all his milestones at the right times or earlier. I recall the sense of relief when I would play my own little game with him. I'd go into the kitchen and call out his name to see if he would turn his head in my direction. What a relief when he'd respond immediately! He was in *our* world.

Watching Connor develop, I realized what it should have been like with Hannah, but wasn't. Connor would usually cry only when he was hungry or wet, and he would definitely let you know when he was ready to get out of his crib. He never had trouble transitioning through the different stages of foods. Unlike Hannah, he would not stay in his bouncy seat very long without flipping it over. He would watch videos for ten minutes on television, and then he was done. He crawled early, sat up early, pulled up early, and walked early. His instinct was to stay with us—unlike Hannah, who wanted to run away without thinking of the consequences of being lost. Connor picked up on things just by watching others—immersion and osmosis—whereas Hannah didn't even notice what other people were doing. Connor pointed at objects and tried to get our attention.

I can remember teaching Hannah to scoop food in her spoon, brush her own hair and teeth, wash herself in the bathtub, dress herself, potty train, tie a shoe, and even peel a banana. Hannah literally had to be directly taught, step by step, everything she knows how to do—things needed to be broken down as if in the game of Candyland. Connor just picked it up. Connor was popping popcorn in the microwave without any help whatsoever before Hannah even knew where the microwave was located. These differences continue to astonish me, but it's Connor's social skills and ability to understand others' perspectives that stand out the most.

At ten years old, Connor is outgoing, articulate, and mature for his age. He has a huge heart and is sensitive to others' needs—and always has been. Even when he was a kindergartener, he would walk around the class helping students read passages and spell words. Part of this is how he was made—hardwired into his personality. But part of it, I think, has come from having a sister who has autism. He's learned to read moods, adjust, accommodate, and make concessions. And he does this with others, reading his friends' moods—and his mom's— and making allowances. He just finished fourth grade in a High Ability classroom with many of his friends. The school had clustered students into cohorts according to aptitude and achievement testing, which placed them together following kindergarten. His friends, along with their families, have been a huge support system for us. Connor thrives in math, reading, speech and debate forums and enjoys participating in Boy Scouts and our church's after school youth group. He also desires to earn his black belt in tae kwon do this year. When hanging out at home, he tinkers with his LEGOs, plays Minecraft on his iPod, and reads action novels like *Percy Jackson*.

We've made an effort to invest in his interests as we get hints of what they might be. Even though he's tagged along on his sister's outings—and they've almost always outnumbered his, especially when he was little—Connor gets to enjoy activities, clubs, and a wonderful group of friends that are his and his alone. That's key. Siblings need a life of their own to avoid being overshadowed by the necessary appointments and medical visits of their brother or sister who has autism. They deserve more than our leftovers. Don't shortchange your typical children.

TWELVE IMPORTANT NEEDS OF SIBLINGS[8]

❖ Siblings need communication that is open, honest, developmentally appropriate, and ongoing.

❖ Siblings need developmentally appropriate and ongoing information about their sibling's ASD.

❖ Siblings need parental attention that is consistent, individualized, and celebrates their uniqueness.

❖ Siblings need time with a parent that is specifically for them. Schedule special time with the sibling on a regular basis.

❖ Siblings need to learn interaction skills with their brother or sister with ASD.

❖ Siblings need choices about how involved they are with their brother or sister.

❖ Siblings need to feel that they and their belongings are safe from their brother or sister with autism.

❖ Siblings need to feel that their brother or sister is being treated as "normal" as possible.

❖ Siblings need time to work through their feelings with patience, understanding, and guidance from their parent(s) and or a professional, if appropriate.

❖ Siblings need opportunities to experience a "normal" family life and activities.

❖ Siblings need opportunities to feel that they are not alone and that others understand and share some of the same experiences.

❖ Siblings need to learn strategies for dealing with questions and comments from peers and others in the community.

SIBLING SUPPORTS

As a parent of a child with autism, your patience, acceptance, and adjustment to your family's situation will be the most important influence on the sibling's experience of having a brother or sister with autism. In other words, our typical children will follow our lead. So I've used several supportive strategies with Connor along our journey.

FORTHRIGHT COMMUNICATION

Connor has been raised always knowing his sister has autism. There have always been therapists in and out of our home. Until Connor understood the reason behind Hannah's extra playmates, which is how I referred to her therapists, I did sense a little jealousy. Periodically, I would make sure Connor was included in the therapy. Otherwise, this was also an opportune time for me to get some one-on-one time with him.

When explaining autism to Connor, I first just told him that Hannah's brain works differently. When he got a little older, I showed him the back of our television. We then followed each cord's specific pathway. I told him the cords' pathways were like his brain. I then asked him to imagine that all of the cords' pathways got mixed up and arrived at the wrong destinations. I told him that was how Hannah's brain felt sometimes. We also read books that were specifically written for siblings of brothers and sisters with autism (see Suggested Resources in the appendix for titles).

Hannah has certain autism-related behaviors that have the ability to inflict anxiety on Connor and me. Sometimes both of us feel as though we must tiptoe around a few of her rituals to make it easier on ourselves. I've tried to help Connor understand how some of her practices are hardwired and although it may not seem like it, she's working desperately to control these behaviors. Connor senses his sister's anxiety all too often in social situations. While playing the Farkle dice game, he'll help her strategize when she's behind because each move presents too many variables for her to have efficient motor planning. While I can't say situations always play out this nicely, there's a warmth in my heart when they do!

ADJUSTING FOR EMOTIONS

We really do try to be normal with inclusive activities, but unfortunately, sometimes the autism still kills it, and there are tears. When playing baseball in the side yard, time after time, if the white plastic ball doesn't come in contact with the oversized gray plastic bat, everyone is sure to be miserable. Once in a while, Connor is the best one to repair the emotional damage Hannah inflicts upon herself after a meltdown. To hear his mature, nurturing, and responsible tone as he soothes her anxiety helps me grow in respect and admiration for all he is becoming. There were also days after school when I'd walk into the house and tell Connor that Hannah's had a bad day at school. He'd ask, "Is she still in the car?" When I said yes, he would head straight out the door to comfort her. That's when I saw a love and understanding oozing from that young man that's bigger than all of us put together.

While Connor understands that it's more challenging for his sister to control her behaviors, he also knows that she will have consequences for them. I don't want Connor to believe it's okay for his sister to misbehave because she has autism, nor do I want to reinforce the destructive behavior for Hannah by not following up with a consequence. As a result, Hannah is held accountable for her destructive behaviors.

Connor does realize that Hannah did not ask for autism or choose autism; it's just how she was made. On Hannah's bad days, I commiserate with him, though we in no way speak disrespectfully about Hannah. Instead, we discuss how hard it is for both of us. Connor often wishes that Hannah would take an interest in and try to understand him. After all, Connor is his sister's most loyal supporter. I suppose I wish she would do the same. I have to believe that she'll take more of an interest in trying to understand both of us one day; in the meantime, her brother is growing in unconditional love and empathy—gifts Hannah has no idea she's giving her brother.

Every human being is different, so not every sibling will respond with as much grace and generosity as Connor. I still remember the first time we met with Hannah's Medicaid caseworker. Connor met her in our home's entry and asked if she could help us with Hannah's difficult behaviors. You can borrow some of my strategies with siblings who are having different reactions to their brother or sister who has autism. If you show a younger child how wires get crossed, perhaps she'll better understand her sibling's struggles. If you set aside special time for your typical child or children when your child with autism is busy with therapy, perhaps they will grow more and more trusting that they are deeply loved. You can also look for your other child(ren)'s strengths and find roles for them to play that make a difference in the family unit.

Do I feel sorry for Connor having to struggle with the environment Hannah sometimes sets? Of course. But I also know that I do an awful lot for my children and try my best to be a good mother. When does my heart hurt the most for my son? When his sister steals his moments to shine. For example, Hannah has a very hard time allowing anyone else in the room other than herself to be complimented. When I compliment Connor, Hannah believes I am simultaneously criticizing her. As a result, I get backlash from her when I praise Connor in her presence. These self-centered thoughts are hard to redirect. We're working on it. I continually remind her that compliments to Connor are not insults directed at her. Connor's successes are not Hannah's failures. Connor says that Hannah puts lemons in his "lime light." She's going to have to improve, because Connor will have a lot of things in his future that will make him stand out, including his sense of humor.

Not long ago, after having a meltdown, Hannah asked Connor, "Do you love me?"

Connor responded, "Hannah, I do love you. But it's a complicated love, not a type of love that you make easy."

PARENTAL ATTENTION

Typical siblings also need and deserve quality time with their parents. Ideally, this time needs to be consistent, individualized, and should recognize their unique interests. I can't compare the time that I need to spend with Hannah to the time I spend with Connor. Hannah does monopolize more time—there's no way around it. Hannah's teachers would say I'm a helicopter parent—a mother hen, while Connor's teachers would say that I'm involved and interested, but more of a hands-off parent. We have to give each child what they need. Good parenting doesn't look the same with each of our children, so we personalize because no child should be overlooked.

Connor and I have our own special times that we cherish. We read chapter books together—to date, we've read almost one hundred. In the evenings before he goes to bed, "Ain't No Mountain High Enough" is our song. We have a special goodbye—an I Love You hand signal known only to us.

I recognize Connor's accomplishments as equally as his sister's, proudly framing his oratorical and tae kwon do certificates, just as I do Hannah's artwork. Self-esteem is directly correlated to positive recognition from parents. Praise and reward your child with autism for each step of progress, and then be sure to praise the typical sibling's expected accomplishments.

SAFETY FOR TYPICAL SIBLINGS AND THEIR BELONGINGS

Siblings must feel they are protected both physically and emotionally in their own home. Some children with autism will push, hit, bite, or engage in other challenging behaviors. Hannah used to be notorious for kicking her brother or others when she became so agitated that she didn't take the time to motor plan her words. Any time this happened, there was an immediate consequence for Hannah and the two were separated. Connor's emotions were always acknowledged and validated. Parents should arrange for and allow typical siblings a safe space for retreat from their sibling's destructive behaviors and also to arrange for safe storage of important items that they don't want taken or destroyed. Destructive behaviors could also take the form of bullying, so watch for it, as this shouldn't be tolerated either. At this stage of their development, I would never leave the two of my kids alone together unsupervised.

SIBLINGS NEED TO EXPERIENCE NORMAL

Don't feel uncomfortable or shy asking for help or utilizing respite care services to look after your child with autism. Draw on community resources and implement Medicaid's autism waiver services. Medicaid is a federal and state medical assistance program that makes reimbursements for reasonable and necessary medical care to people meeting eligibility requirements. Respite care services, provided by Medicaid, provide temporary relief to those unpaid persons normally providing care. With the autism waiver, some of your parental duties qualify you as the unpaid caregiver and allow you to receive support. Contact your state's family and social services agency for information on the application process.

Though these experiences are bittersweet in that you realize you cannot enjoy all experiences together as a family, typical siblings and parents need opportunities for activities where the focus and energy is not at all directed toward the child with autism. Don't deny your typical child activities outside of the home either! Find some way for them to participate in sports, clubs, gatherings—maybe carpool, ask your spouse (or ex-spouse), or contact the activity's sponsor. Remember, you are reaching out in order for your child to have an opportunity—feel no guilt in that. Also keep in mind that it is not the typical child's job to watch over their sibling.

ISOLATED FEELINGS AND EXPLANATIONS TO FRIENDS

Connor knows that I try to make everything seem normal, but we both know it's not. Connor tolerates a lot of unpleasant behaviors and time-consuming activities associated with Hannah, and sometimes I forget how truly hard it must be on him. He knows this is how it has to be with her—even as he frequently questions how she could only care about herself. In his own words, Connor says that *Hannah's autism is the way it has to be, but that doesn't mean it doesn't suck a little.* Hannah's starting to try to understand her brother's and my feelings more, but **cognitive empathy** is not one of her strengths.

Typical siblings need opportunities to share their feelings and emotions with other kids in similar situations and with grown adults who have already navigated autism's nuances with their families. They need to know they're not alone and that others understand and share some of the same experiences. These opportunities are so valuable. Look to see if your area has a sibling support group or offers sibling events. Online resources such as Sibshops (SibNet and SibTeen) are also available.

Brothers and sisters with a sibling on the spectrum should also be guided with an approach to feel comfortable when discussing their sibling's autism with friends. They need to learn strategies for answering questions and dealing with comments from others who don't understand the disability. As parents, it's our job to prepare our typical children for possible reactions from others toward their sibling with autism. We also need to understand that there may be a time when they're embarrassed by their sibling on the spectrum. These are real feelings that should be softly addressed without criticism, followed by generating possible solutions. If there is someone available to watch Hannah during Connor's activities, I make that happen.

When Connor has friends over, I try to either keep Hannah busy or have her stay with someone else to allow Connor uninterrupted time with his friends. I know Connor appreciates this gesture.

NO SIBLINGS IN THE SHADOWS

I've seen terminology used for typical siblings who have a sibling on the spectrum, and they make me cringe. These terms include *collateral damage*, *autism's invisible victims*, and *the forgotten ones*. As parents, we can't allow this to happen. A friend of mine attended a sibling panel at an autism conference in which the animosity of the siblings toward their situations was painful and insulting. She walked out in tears. If we as parents remain aware of the pitfalls and seek to see from our typical child's perspective, we might be able to alleviate this attitude. Maybe not, but we certainly don't want to add to it. We cannot guarantee a happy outcome, but we can take measures to encourage flexibility, forgiveness, understanding, and individuality that hopefully give all our typical children a positive view of their sibling on the spectrum—and their own childhood years.

WORDS OF CAUTION FOR TYPICAL SIBLINGS

The pros and cons of growing up with a sibling on the spectrum will present gifts and challenges, as you can see. Let me offer a few final words of caution for typical siblings—and for you, as the parent.

MATURE BEYOND THEIR YEARS

Siblings with a brother or sister on the spectrum have experienced a reality that has made the concerns and worries of other children who are the same age seem minuscule. They've had to grow up faster by helping around the house, being more independent, and witnessing the challenges of their brother or sister with autism daily. While maturity is beneficial, make sure you and your typical child don't miss out on their childhood.

DRIVEN FOR SUCCESS

It's no surprise that typical siblings tend to aspire to achieve at high levels outside of the home.[9] I see this in Connor. They often believe they possess more of a voice outside of the home than inside. However, they sometimes believe they must compensate for their sibling's deficit in order to prove to their parents that they're good at parenting. If this is the case, this belief must be squelched. And while we must find safe places and people to be honest with about our parenting doubts and struggles, be careful what you say in front of your children. They must do well in order to be proud of themselves, not to make up for their sibling's challenges. As the typical child or children grow older, be careful not to turn to him or her as a confidante, confessing your concerns about your child on the spectrum. They need you to be their parent, so don't speak with them as a friend seeking support or advice.

CONCERNS FOR THE FUTURE

Many typical brothers and sisters worry about future obligations. Will they have to care for their sibling with autism if something should happen to their parents? Communicate clearly that they will be afforded the right to their own lives. Make sure they have your blessing to pursue their dreams, and assure them any future involvement with their sibling on the spectrum will be a choice, not an obligation. Siblings' attitudes toward the extent of their involvement may also change over time. Do not place the burden of a decision on young children or even teens.

FIVE BENEFITS OF GROWING UP WITH AN AUTISTIC SIBLING[10]

* Perception: Having an autistic sibling means growing up alongside someone who sees the world in a unique, individual way—a way that is often different from the mainstream population.

* Perspective: Growing up with an autistic sibling means watching your sibling face each day with more courage and strength than most of us can fathom.

* Leadership: Siblings of autistic children often have to mature very early—arguably, earlier than should be required. By necessity, siblings often must assist their parents in helping, providing care, and teaching.

* Courage: By necessity, growing up with an autistic sibling teaches a child to have the courage to stand out.

* Creativity: Many of the other listed benefits have underlying tones of creativity, or produce creativity as a byproduct of the other attributes achieved.

A SIBLING PANEL

In the summer of 2015 I was able to sit in on a sibling panel break-out session at the Autism Society of America's national conference in Denver. Led by auto racing's Jason Cherry (founder of Siblings of Autism), their words were genuine and comforting—hope for my son. The five typical siblings from different families, all around the age of twenty-five, said they were brothers and sisters trying to cope with one another, and that the outbursts were very hard. They said that sometimes they just had to laugh with their family after a situation because they didn't want to spend the rest of their life crying. They definitely noticed a maturity difference in school between themselves and their peers and believe their brother or sister's autism taught them not to judge people and to think outside of themselves.

Each sibling agreed that they were staunch advocates for the larger autism community. They each showed an understanding of their siblings and their siblings' autism, which revealed their character. No matter how far out their siblings' ideas were, they always supported them. They said they were so good at reading their siblings that all they had to do was look at them and they could tell what was going to happen.

They agreed they had an idealism that they could change the world—perhaps in part because they have already faced so much and seen their siblings change over the years—and all of them excelled outside of the home.

A FINAL WORD ON BEHALF OF TYPICAL SIBLINGS

Fostering good relationships between siblings takes love, patience, and time. We can't force our kids to have good relationships, but we can facilitate opportunities for them to play together and find common interests. I try to structure some activities that include areas of interest for Hannah and Connor and provide support and communication or behavioral aids when necessary. We're coming along. Connor doesn't think his sister cares for him, but I know differently.

A typical sibling can influence his or her sibling with autism in significant ways. Connor may be two years younger than Hannah, but he's been Hannah's *typically developing role model*. He will be in his sister's life longer than his father and me or any service provider; though he will never be obligated to be his sister's keeper, their futures are inexorable entwined. As parents, we need to do our absolute best to make sure our attention is vested in each of our children—typical and on the spectrum.

Typical siblings will also learn how to be there for you—like Connor already has for me. They develop the skills and attitude to be great advocates not only for their brother or sister, but for the entire special needs community. One evening after the kids had gone to bed, I was downstairs watching the television show *Parenthood*. Connor couldn't sleep, so he came downstairs with a book and read while I continued watching the show. One of show's storylines follows the Braverman family as they navigate the journey of Max, a character with Asperger's syndrome—the reason I make time to watch a television show. With-out my saying a word, Connor looked at me and said, "Everything has to be perfect for that Max kid, just like Hannah." Yes, I see shades of Max in Hannah.

We'll spend so much of our lives speaking up for our child with autism—let's speak up for our typical children, too. They need us to be proactive in helping them, so they don't get lost in the shuffle. They need a chance to shine.

I am so lucky I get to be Connor's mother. When he shines, I'm glowing with joy.

Wisdom from the Round Table

Lori R.: We have three other children besides Cameron. My daughter, now twenty-one, has always been like a second mother to Cameron. She did a week-long blog about what life was like having a sibling with autism. The blog raised funds for Riley Children's Hospital. There have been times when my kids have been embarrassed by Cameron's behavior, but that's normal. They've been embarrassed by their other siblings' behavior too!

Jen: I always wanted four children. After Noah's autism diagnosis, we contemplated having another child, and then we decided to put it into God's hands. Noah is an only child.

Lori V.: I tried, to the best of my ability, to give enough time to our other son, Devin. I allowed him to pursue his interests and enjoy them. Sometimes I would need to take Byron with me, and this would mean that much of the time trying to *be there* for Devin meant tending to his brother's needs at the event. Sometimes my thinly veiled exhaustion bordered on insanity. Devin did feel awkward with Byron in public around the age of sixteen and seventeen. When peers accepted Byron, then he felt it was okay. After high school graduation, I was adamant that Devin live on a college campus. He needed to get away from it all.

Susan: I've never seen anyone with as much compassion for special needs children as I have seen with Allie. I can remember so many times that Allie and I would be on the bed crying while Tyler would bang on the bedroom door. There were times I would yell at Allie just because I was so frustrated with Tyler's behavior. Allie had to grow up a lot faster than other children her age. She has seen and experienced more things in her young life than her peers have ever seen or experienced. I hate that!

While it's hard to look back on those times, she is confident, strong, and independent. But I always play the "what if . . ." game with both Ty and Allie. I felt guilty as a mom that Allie never knew what normal was like. What am I saying? I don't even know what normal is like. Others are sad when their children go off to college. I was so thrilled for Allie. She was finally going to know normal.

Karen: Both of my boys do have autism, and they shape one another. John is orderly and unbelievably stubborn, even more stubborn than I am, and that has taught Eric to be careful how he lays out plans. Eric is disorganized and impulsive, and that has taught John some flexibility. The boys are good at helping one another see from a different perspective. They complement and understand one another.

Sarah: Mitchell's sister is eighteen months younger than he is. She has always done more around the house and felt it not fair. She's significantly more mature than her older brother and treated as such. When we told her about his autism diagnosis, a light went on for her. Now she has compassion for him. The reality is that our youngest son hasn't gotten as much attention as I would like because of Mitchell's autism.

CHAPTER SIX

strength in numbers

The Power of Community

For a parent that is living with their child's diagnosis of autism, it's all about community. Community is everything!

—John Donvan

September 2008

Today we're not only participating in the Answers for Autism Walk, like last year, but we've formed Hannah's Team! I glance at the sky— not a single cloud drifting over the park. We unload Hannah (three and a half years old) and Connor (one and a half years old), and I grab the green umbrella stroller. The sides of Hannah's hair are pulled back in French braids and tied together with a bright yellow ribbon. Despite the huge adjustment to her Saturday schedule, Hannah sure is in a good mood. We begin to search the parking lot for our family and friends.

My friend's parents own a printing company and designed our team shirts for our family's big day. They're yellow—Hannah's favorite color. As I scan the parking lot and park itself, the event's venue, I am shocked to see a sea of yellow covers the park—apparently, this year's event shirt happens to be the same color I chose for Hannah's Team shirts. Of all the colors to choose this year!

After we corral Hannah's Team, I look around at all of these friends and family members gathered for one reason—to support our family. Over forty people join us from all different walks of our life. We easily surpassed our lofty first-time fundraising and participation goals.

Large activity tents offer sensory-friendly opportunities to engage in family fun! Hannah runs from table to table seeking different experiences. We all follow for fear of losing her in the mass of yellow. First, she runs to a table where kids are rubbing shaving cream all over the table's surface. Her hypersensitivity to touch alerts her. The look on her face reads, I'm getting out of here. *Next, she walks over yards and yards of bubble wrap—appreciating the sensory input. She finds a craft table where a volunteer gestures for her to make a puzzle piece frame. She dodges the volunteer because she eyes several inflated baby pools filled with brightly colored plastic balls. She methodically maneuvers herself one of the pools and enjoys the experience until another child jumps in to join her.*

I quickly lift her out of the pool, and she dashes to a table with musical instruments. If given a choice, she would remain here the rest of the day. She becomes fixated on a large, thin, hand-held white drum and clings to it, thumping in a steady rhythm with the mallet. The emcee is summoning everyone to the stage area, but Hannah isn't going to let go of the drum or mallet without a fight. She hugs it and turns away from me. I try to coax her to put it down, hoping she won't put a damper on Hannah's Team by throwing a dramatic fit. Thankfully, a volunteer allows us to keep the instrument and return it after the walk. I say "thank you" over and over.

The emcee on the stage introduces one of the entertainers, Braden Daniels, who sings the walk's annual kick-off song, "I Wouldn't Have It Any Other Way." The song echoes every parent's journey with autism: the dream to understand and reach our children, intense frustration with not knowing what to do, and, most poignantly, our unconditional love and acceptance.

My mother brings a hand to her face to gently wipe a tear while a friend uses her yellow sleeve. All forty of us are sighing or looking at each other through blurry eyes, trying to control our emotions.

The entire crowd, awash with tethered yellow balloons, recites the autism balloon release poem. The releasing of the balloons symbolizes our support in helping individuals with autism remove all barriers, so they can soar to their highest potential. The sky is now filled with yellow acceptance and advocacy. I turn from the balloons to Hannah. She's smiling as she watches the mass of yellow rising above her. I so rarely see that smile.

Our team gathers for a short prayer, then we find a place on the paved trail to walk. At the last minute, my assistant principal shows up with our school's office staff—more friends!—and they're giddy with excitement. We're laughing and Hannah is standing among us all, anxiety-free.

The walk commences at a snail's pace, and Hannah is still wearing the same smile that has continued to brighten everyone's morning. Connor finds his place on top of his daddy's shoulders, and then in my friend Lori's arms. He's becoming such a big boy. Hannah takes turns walking with different people, thumping her borrowed drum. After half a mile, she climbs into the green stroller. Everyone has respected her sensitivity to touch, but she's ready to take it easy. I don't think she has any idea that everyone in our group is here celebrating her! That's okay, though, because I know.

The rolling green landscape, mirroring ponds, stately bridge, and twin bell towers provide a picturesque and elegant venue for such a momentous event. As we stroll through the Children's Garden, I notice a sign that reads DRAGONFLY ISLAND. *It's designed to resemble its given name.*

As we cross the finish line, we all lower our heads to receive our medal. Now, Hannah has something new to fascinate on, and this is my chance to return the drum.

Today, I don't feel different. Today, I feel proud and at peace, knowing my little girl is loved and autism is accepted.

When a family receives a diagnosis of autism, they usually feel isolated—as though they no longer fit into the same society. We did. I felt as if I were wearing a scarlet letter. I thought it was necessary to tell everyone that my daughter had autism. Although this feeling was only temporary, it was real. As I shared our status over and over—even with strangers—I was searching for others who were like us.

I'd share with our community's librarian while checking out books about autism, and I'd hear, "Have they ever found out what causes that?"

I'd share with a fellow greeter at our church, and I'd hear, "Oh, I'm sorry . . . that must be hard."

I'd share at back-to-school night with another parent whose child was in Hannah's class, and I'd hear, "You really can't tell by looking at her that she has autism. I never would've known. It's good she can be in a normal class."

I'm even sure I considered going door-to-door around our cul-de-sac making sure each person knew our situation.

At the time, I didn't know what I expected or wanted to receive by continuing to do this. It wasn't pity. At times it felt like I needed to confess a family secret. But in the end, I kept sharing because I needed to know I wasn't alone. I longed for stories and solutions from people who *understood*. I craved the company of those whose plight and challenges were similar. I wanted to find a community of people locally and virtually who were familiar with all things autism.

The good news is . . . I found them. And while I don't recommend you take my approach and tell every waiter or grocery store cashier you interact with that your daughter or son has autism, you will find your people who understand. And you'll find them in all kinds of places, even on a short commute in a taxi from the airport to the beach.

Autism doesn't have to be isolating because as you'll soon see, it's all about community, and families will find many opportunities where they'll feel accepted and supported. It's amazing when community, passion, and real-life responsibilities collide in such a meaningful way. Seeing other moms and dads embrace autism gave me strength to carry on day after day, and more importantly, it awakened in me a deeper love for Hannah. In time, the solidarity I experienced with others led me to a role bigger than I ever imagined: I felt called to become an advocate for all of those with autism, and what an amazing mission!

COMMUNITY OPPORTUNITIES

I've grown to appreciate the virtual network of support I've developed with people all over the nation, and I cherish my long-distance friends, but nothing beats meeting with people in person, locally. You can find other families who have children with autism at a variety of community events and gatherings.

AUTISM WALKS

I'll never forget our family's first autism walk. Hannah had just been diagnosed, and Connor was around six months old. I had doubts and was very apprehensive about our participation. We were still new to the diagnosis, feeling raw and vulnerable. I knew we would know no one and wondered if the event would thicken our blanket of grief.

All my worries were alleviated as soon as we arrived. The atmosphere was festive and inviting. People were happy! Bounce houses, sensory stations, and excitement filled the park. During the walk, I heard laughter all around me and marveled at the joy. Was this what a world with autism could feel like? Even after back-to-back appointments, brutal schedules, meltdowns, and misunderstandings? I felt as if I'd entered an alternate universe.

This was our first positive event related to autism—it gave us hope and energy to meet the challenges we faced in our home. The walk served as a wonderful metaphor for us—that we don't have to walk this road alone. Every family has to figure out how they will structure their day-to-day lives, but we don't have to walk through life isolated. All around us are families who can laugh and cry and problem-solve with us.

Look for an event like this walk, which is a state walk. Other states hold similar events. You can also join the Autism Speaks Walk, the world's largest autism fundraising event dedicated to improving the lives of people with autism. They're sure to have a walk near you! See the Suggested Resources section for more information.

AUTISM SUPPORT GROUPS

Families coping with autism's challenges need an outlet where they can unload their concerns. Contrary to how we may feel on any given day, we are not left alone to deal with trials specific to only our family. We can gather in local support groups with other parents who are going through the same things.

Because parents with typical children may not understand the unique issues we face, the support group setting works well. To hear others describe challenges—even anguish—similar to ours makes us feel as if we are not alone. The first time I heard other parents describe meltdowns, sensory disorders, eating challenges, and ritualistic behaviors like we were facing with Hannah, I felt a strange comfort. I knew I had resources surrounding me. I asked questions about how they would solve a particular problem we were having with her auditory sensitivity, and several people gave us strategies to try. Over time, I learned enough to provide newcomers with the same kind of problem-solving input.

These meetings are not what I'd call fun, but I think you'll leave them a lot lighter because you'll have shared true feelings with others who listen without judgment or scorn. People are actually nodding their heads and validating your experiences. They understand the new vocabulary and medical terminology that has all of a sudden been added to your lexicon. It was difficult, however, when others who were further along on the journey discussed challenging milestones that we couldn't bear to come to grips with yet, such as the dire question, "Who will take care of my child when I am gone?" I still believe, though, the support and understanding that you receive outweigh the fearful topics suggested.

MENTORS

When Hannah was first diagnosed, our area also had a program called Family-to-Family that provided services to families in a variety of ways. We were assigned a parent liaison whose job was to provide us with extensive resource materials in the areas of health insurance, special education law, community resources, trainings, and support organizations. A decade later, thanks to autism awareness and advocacy, many states have their own Autism Society of America affiliate chapter, which has streamlined the search for a variety of resources and needs.

Our family was also matched with two parent mentors from different families who had recently traveled through the same developmental milestones as those we were heading into with Hannah. Through this program we found our parent support group and special activities held for families with a child on the spectrum. Although neither of these relationships flourished past a few years, both fit our needs at a specific point along our journey. Believe me, where you are today will not be the same place you'll be tomorrow. Find what you need right now and trust that the next person or group will be there when you need something different.

We also reached out to the Indiana Resource Center for Autism located at Indiana University. The center's director, Dr. Cathy Pratt, is a specialist in the field. She met with our family and gave suggestions for Hannah. You can search for similar experts at nearby universities and hospitals to see if they can answer specific concerns and questions.

LONG-DISTANCE AND VIRTUAL COMMUNITY

If you live in a small town or rural setting, or if you have specialized concerns that your local resources and community can't address, reach further out to resources with national recognition and online spokespeople, advocates, and experts.

NATIONAL AUTISM CONFERENCES

Along our autism journey, I have found there is a right time to do everything. I wasn't ready to attend my first national conference until July 2015. Before then, I was too busy surviving and worrying about Hannah's daily rigid routine and schedule to be able to see autism on a larger scale in a public forum. By the summer of 2015, Hannah responded well to other caregivers who kept her on her predictable schedule, so I made my first big travel plans.

I obtained a grant, or I couldn't have afforded to attend the Autism Society's national conference and exposition in Denver, Colorado. If you're dealing with limited funds and your child is younger, begin your search for available grants by contacting your state's early intervention program. I was upset with myself about missing out on that opportunity. Because Hannah is older, grant money is available through the autism Medicaid waiver for our family.

For those few days, I was steeped in the most current findings and methodology in the field of autism research, listening to presentations from researchers, parents, authors, counselors, and adults who themselves had autism. I took copious notes as I immersed myself in both the keynote content and the messages by speakers leading breakout sessions. I made a point to ask specific questions to directly help Hannah. Don't be shy at these events! I met all the keynote speakers and breakout session speakers either before or after their presentations, mingling with educators and parents alike. Believe me, if you don't take the opportunity when it presents itself, you'll find yourself upset when you return home. I spoke with Temple Grandin and reminded her of our first encounter years before when I drove to Evansville, Indiana, to hear her speak. I met Jennifer O'Toole and listened to David Finch, Michelle Garcia Winner, and Chloe Rothschild. I was also excited to meet Sharon Cummings and her son, Conner, who are responsible for enacting Conner's Law in the state of Virginia. Sharon is also the co-founder, publisher, and executive director of *Zoom*, a digital magazine focusing on autism through many lenses. A vendor shared a hint that resources are generally discounted on the last day, so I waited until the last day at the expo to purchase resources.

Temple Grandin reinforced the importance of job skills for kids on the spectrum. She also discussed the value of allowing kids with autism to explore their special interests. Jennifer O'Toole gave the audience tools to strengthen communication with children with autism. The next day she led a discussion by the *Sisterhood of the Spectrum* panel. These were females with autism who were featured in her book *Sisterhood of the Spectrum: An Asperger Chick's Guide to Life*. David Finch, author of *The Journal of Best Practices*, explained why it's so difficult for kids with autism to pay attention in a regular classroom without accommodations and/or modifications. A speech-language pathologist, Michelle Garcia Winner, discussed social cognitive deficits, while Chloe Rothschild, young adult with autism and advocate, discussed her challenges with receptive, expressive, and social communication. It would take me years to glean from books and podcasts the same amount of content I absorbed in the three days I was in Colorado. The pace was intense—this was no restful mountain retreat. But the content was gold.

I enjoyed the entire conference, but I realized as I reflected on the event during my flight home that my favorite part of all was the meet-and-greet the Wednesday evening prior to the conference. Unbeknownst to me, most of the attendees at that particular session had Asperger's syndrome. I was in the exact element I yearned for—these people handed me a crystal ball to peer into Hannah's future. I told them that my daughter had Asperger's syndrome, and that I was also a teacher and taught students with autism who were mainstreamed into my classroom. "What can you tell me to help my daughter and my students?" I asked. They discussed the advantages, challenges, and need for sensory breaks and gave me ideas like integrating more technology to aid with communication. They shared that if Hannah can find a place where she can relax and unwind, that we should cherish it and use it! This got me going: I fired off question after question, and they were so quick and adamant with their answers.

"How can I help with faster transitions and specific materials needed for classes?"

"Don't have them use a locker, allow a backpack in class, and tape a schedule and list of materials to the front of their binder."

"What about a child in class that needs to process information at one hundred percent or he'll continue asking questions that diminish the class's rigor?"

"Allow him a certain number of questions determined by the number of chips you give him. After the chips have all been returned to you, he's to write his questions in a notebook or see you during downtime. Then, using his affinities, create a scenario in his mind where he's trying to teach students something specific about his affinity, and one individual continues to ask more of the same questions. His lesson about his affinity won't get completed. Thus, he's able to see the situation he's causing in his point of view."

We continued the volleys for at least twenty minutes. They taught me so much that evening. This was worth the price of admission, and I hadn't even sat through the first keynote address!

A man named Jean shared with me that a minimized schedule on his computer is of the utmost of importance for him because of a lack of executive functioning skills. Verbal directions or lists continue to be a challenge for him. His sensory challenges make it necessary to rate clothes on how long he is able to bear them being on him like a second skin.

Another man, Carl, shared with me that he chose computer programming for his career because he can count on one hand the number of people he has to talk to in one day—the solitary nature of this work means he chooses his interactions. He called it self-preservation. He then recalled the pleasant sensory experience he has on the way home from work, feeling the air across his face as he rides on his motorcycle. "Home is a safe place for me," he said, "after I've had to hold it together all day."

More individuals with autism shared their ideas with me. When I asked a man named Jeff about Hannah's eye contact, he said, "You can tell me to look at you or listen to you; however, we are going to tangle if you tell me to do both." He said that his honesty still gets in the way. Jeff stopped me when I told him that Hannah had high-functioning autism. "General euphemisms are quite offensive," he explained, urging me to be careful about repeating Hannah's label because the label is only to be used for understanding her behaviors. And he said meltdowns can only be controlled by understanding their antecedents (triggers), and they are the last resort for a child with autism.

This level of detailed input from the broader community available, briefly, once a year is priceless. These interactions provided solid evidence for how strength in numbers can change the way we view our world as families dealing with autism.

I attended the same conference the following year in New Orleans. They offered a special screening of *Life, Animated*—a movie adapted from Ron Suskind's book about his son, Owen, with autism. Ron held a discussion after the movie that verified my thoughts that our children's affinities could be our passport into their worlds.

That year I met Steve Silberman, author of *Neurotribes*; Susan Senator, author of *Making Peace with Autism: One Family's Story of Struggle, Discovery, and Unexpected Gifts*; Barry Prizant, author of

Uniquely Human; James Ball, author of *Early Intervention and Autism: Real-Life Answers, Real-Life Questions;* Stephen Shore, author of *Beyond the Wall: Personal Experiences with Autism and Asperger Syndrome;* and John Donvan and Caren Zucker, co-authors of *In a Different Key: The Story of Autism.* Michael Tolleson, a famous savant autist, was kind enough to paint a dragonfly on canvas for Hannah. All of these people, gathered together to form a rich community. They enlighten parents on our child's emotions, needs, and authentic self more than I could ever dream of doing. Seek out these resources: they will be invaluable in making the journey with your child.

I cannot stress the level of professionalism, outreach, and courtesy I've enjoyed each time I've attended a national conference. While both were sponsored by the Autism Society of America, each conference had a different overall feel and focus that I didn't anticipate leading into the next.

Several national conferences are held throughout the year. Research to find the one that best aligns with your philosophies and developmental stage. You can review the theme, keynote topics, and breakout sessions to see if enough content will be applicable. And, as I mentioned, I didn't attend one of these long-distance events until Hannah was in upper elementary school. Choose the right time for yourself so you aren't overwhelmed leaving your child or children at home with others.

WEBSITES AND BLOGS

The all-consuming nature of being a single working mom with two children—one of whom has autism—limits my free time. I spend very little of it on my computer doing anything other than course or curriculum planning and grading. In fact, I've only been on Facebook since the fall of 2015, and I can't remember the last time I allowed myself the luxury of watching an entire television show. However, after reading Kelle Hampton's book *Bloom,* about her daughter Ella's diagnosis of Down syndrome, I decided to check out her blog. I was captivated by her determination to find joy in the small things in life. I decided to see if any parents of children with autism were on the same journey as my family and chronicling it online.

I found many incredible resources, many of them actual people who interact with their readers, and I can see what a gift this virtual community is, especially for parents who have few resources and cannot easily travel. Their presence is available through social media and the content they publish on their websites.

In fact, through Facebook and Twitter, friends are sharing blog posts and articles on autism that are of special interest to me. I subscribe to a lot of them, save their websites as a favorite, or just copy the post URL in Instant Messenger. As I read through each parent's blog post, I'm always thinking, Yes, I know how that feels. Though I have over one hundred books on autism, blogs are different. They're personal and offer a sense of camaraderie, which I look for even online. The bloggers publish quick reads that you don't have to buy and offer a sense of immediacy—I feel like this is what the family is dealing with right here, right now, and that feels fresh and real. They focus on a single topic—a topic that may affirm and explain what I'm seeing in Hannah. I also pick up ideas and techniques from their solution-oriented content to further her independence.

One big reason parents blog is to use that space as a sounding board to tell their stories. Writing is cathartic for them, and they want to hear readers respond to their ideas and stories. I know from personal experience that expressing your innermost emotions in words and recording them on a page makes them seem more real—sharing it all with others gives valuable feedback.

Most of all, blogs are the basis of an online community of parents. Parents with kids who have autism love to blog because this outlet enables community with others. Readers flock to compelling blogs because the author's experiences are well-told variations on their own challenging lives—we see ourselves in the stories a blogger shares, and we feel less alone. The situations are real. Even the best parents face challenging behaviors from their children; blogs that discuss autism's challenges make us feel as though we aren't doing anything wrong as parents. If you haven't subscribed to a blog or two, try it! They don't cost anything but your time. My only concern is to pay attention to your patterns and be sure that blogs don't become a compulsion or add to your grieving.

RECOMMENDED AUTISM WEBSITES AND BLOGS

❖ Autism Society (www.autism-society.org)
❖ Autism Speaks (www.autismspeaks.org)
❖ Carrie Cariello: Exploring the Colorful World of Autism (www.carriecariello.com)
❖ Jason Hague (www.jasonhague.com)
❖ Jennifer O'Toole (www.asperkids.com)
❖ Kerry Magro (www.kerrymagro.com)
❖ Susan Senator (www.susansenator.com)
❖ and my own, Lori Ashley Taylor (www.emergingfromautism.com)

LOCAL COMMUNITY

The online and national gatherings offer incredible experiences, but local events bring people in your own physical community together for far less money and effort than a national event and in a much more intimate setting than you'll experience clicking through articles online.

LOCAL AUTISM WORKSHOPS AND CONFERENCES

I'll never forget my first autism workshop. Hannah had just been diagnosed with autism, and I wasn't yet ready to start delving into anything outside of the immediate therapies she was receiving inside our home. However, that school year, my teaching partners and I had a boy on our academic team diagnosed with Asperger's syndrome. Both of my partners said they wanted to know more about autism in order to help the student as much as possible. I was grieving Hannah's diagnosis at the time and went along with their ploy to learn more about autism not only to help our student, but also to support me.

Local autism workshops give parents, teachers, and therapists the tools we need to help children grow behaviorally and academically. I know there is no one-size-fits-all for autism, but I've never been to a local workshop that was not worth my time and money for my daughter. That first workshop in 2006 defined the categories of autism for me, instructed me on how to make visual schedules and personalized stories, discussed the importance of physical structure of the classroom, outlined organization of learning space, and more. Essentially, they break down large ideas that our children can't fathom into smaller, tangible pieces of information made easier to process.

I've also attended local autism conferences with presentations by Temple Grandin, Eustacia Cutler (Temple Grandin's mother), and Dr. Jed Baker, director of the Social Skills Training Project. Temple Grandin spoke about her sensory-based world. Eustacia Cutler discussed her challenges raising Temple when autism was not accepted by the general population as it is today. She recalled being accused of being a *refrigerator mother,* an appalling term and horrendous reigning psychiatric orthodox of the 1940s, '50s, and '60s coined by Leo Kanner to describe the mothering of children with autism as if from a refrigerator that didn't defrost. What an offensive and erroneous theory! I encourage you to read her book *A Thorn in My Pocket.* Jed Baker discussed effective interventions for behavioral and social challenges. All of these workshops enlightened me to try something different than what I had been doing with Hannah.

Area workshops and conferences are less expensive than the national ones and offer more time on specific subjects. They're also smaller and less overwhelming—and they require less time and fewer resources to attend. Two-day or weekend events are easier to attend if they're in town and you don't have to go away overnight. You can find some organized as one-day seminars, which are easier for moms with young children to attend.

Check out what your local autism organization or coalition has to offer. And don't be afraid to ask about financial assistance—it's there for a reason. It might as well be you that uses it!

LOCAL OPPORTUNITIES FOR YOUR CHILD WITH AUTISM

As autism has become more accepted, opportunities for our children have also expanded. There are quality camps, sensory-friendly film screenings, art exhibitions, gymnastic classes, music classes, and more. Our town has a parenting magazine that always includes special opportunities for children with autism. Find out if your town or city has a magazine that does the same and subscribe to it so you don't miss out on opportunities that suit your child. Your local or state autism association or society may also offer a calendar of events. And, remember, if our children never have opportunities to be in public, they will never acquire the skills needed to be successful outside of their home and school. Helping them build community in their own way, interacting with and responding to social cues, will help them grow to more functional people as they mature.

SCHOOL SYSTEM AUTISM TEAM AND SPECIAL NEEDS MINISTRY

Our school system is always looking for leadership in a variety of areas. After twenty-four years as a classroom teacher, mine used to be in math and science; however, I've found a new niche. I serve on our school system's autism team. This is an opportune way for me to assist in a dual role as parent and teacher. I get to learn firsthand what is affecting our system's autism population the most. I speak on different topics at meetings, serve as a parent resource, help organize our district's autism fair, and try my hardest to understand new screenings and testing. Look for similar teams in your school system and learn all you can from these people who are serving and teaching your child.

I've also found community within the special needs ministry at our church. Growing up in the church, Hannah has always been accepted as she is—autism and all! Although each member of our group has children with different needs, we're all there for one another. There is comfort in our time spent together. We work to spread awareness about our journeys with others in our congregation by speaking annually at our church service. We also provide a time and place for our adults with special needs to gather and enjoy one another's company. Connect with your faith community, if you're part of one, to see what they offer. Or maybe you can propose a simple one-time event to see who else among your membership has children on the spectrum. This group's support has been so helpful during our journey.

COMMUNITY AS SANCTITY

Last year Hannah and I decided that just the two of us would go to our state autism walk. As usual, we first headed to the sensory tent station.

Hannah saw an older boy there, around sixteen years old, who was having a difficult time dipping a bubble wand into the bubble liquid, lifting the wand out of the liquid, and waving it to produce bubbles. Without any prompting, Hannah walked over to the boy and said, "Hi! My name is Hannah. Do you have autism like me? All the steps needed for the bubbles are tricky. Here, watch me. First, dip the entire wand. Then pull the wand out and place it sideways like this at your side. And, lastly, swing the wand as quickly as you can to the other side of your body. See?" Lots of bubbles came out for Hannah. You can tell she's a therapy kid! The boy tried it again with Hannah repeating the steps, and he did it! I looked to see her reaction, and she was smiling. I felt a remarkable lump in my throat.

We benefited from an entire village of skilled people who positively affected our family's life, both close by and far off, in person and online—I hope every family with a child on the spectrum can experience an improved quality of life with similar support. Get involved with autism's wonderful community of people, because they know that sometimes the smallest steps are actually the biggest accomplishments.

✺ Wisdom from the Round Table ✺

Lori R.: Once Cameron was diagnosed, I immersed myself in attending every workshop, conference, training, and support group that I possibly could! It was overwhelming to say the least, but I found strength in numbers. I didn't feel so alone, gained valuable insights, learned how to help my son and family, and I met some pretty amazing people!

Jen: After Noah's diagnosis at age two, I wanted what was best for him, but I never sought out support groups or online blogs. They were too overwhelming, and I was dealing with a diagnosis. I didn't want to hear about anyone else's journey. I went to everything in prayer. God guided us along the journey we needed to take.

Lori V.: Opportunities to connect with parents in similar situations have been a welcome part of my journey. For me, the greatest connection was becoming a parent advocate for parents of children with special needs. I was blessed to be able to get to know two other moms of children on the spectrum. A great kinship evolved with these two women! Also, helping parents who are frustrated and overwhelmed with trying to obtain educational opportunities has helped them and helped me understand that we're all united by common wants and desires for ourselves and our children. We all need to vent and let it go to someone who truly gets it. I also became a tutor for higher-functioning children on the spectrum. Helping them to succeed and teaching them the way they need to learn has brought me more joy and has been so rewarding and comforting for me. These parents and children have become a family to me and we continue to stay in contact. It's a bond that we'll always share.

Susan: Most of the interactions I've had with other families have been through school—either at school organized events or events specifically for special needs children such as Special Olympics and Transition Fairs. With my position as a school psychologist, I've gained a lot of information through my own professional organizations such as Indiana Association of School Psychologists. I was recently asked to serve on the Human Rights Committee for Indiana Mentor, my son Tyler's residential provider.

Karen: When I look back, now twelve years ago, I don't think I relied much on autism community support because my two children are high-functioning. Teachers at school and the occupational and speech therapists were the best resources for us. In late childhood years, a teen behavior and social skills group at the speech therapy department of Riley Children's Hospital was beneficial. Sitting in the waiting room and hearing other parents' stories was a good experience for me.

Sarah: Meeting other parents of kids on the spectrum allowed me to talk through our issues and realize the struggles we had weren't ours alone—there were other people struggling too. It was so helpful to have people I could talk to that would actually understand and not judge the parenting choices we were making just to survive. I've also joined an online group for parents of twice-exceptional children, which has allowed me to gain that same kind of acceptance and camaraderie with parents whose kids are not only challenged with a learning or developmental disability, but who are considered "gifted" intellectually. That in itself is a hard road to navigate, as many teachers, school systems, and even family members struggle to understand how a child can appear simultaneously brilliant and totally clueless. Having a support system of parents who get it helps push aside the loneliness, and also helps with advice on how to best advocate for my child!

CHAPTER SEVEN

changing normal

Stage Two Interventions

Focus more on who your child is than on what your child does.
Remember you're growing a person, not fixing a problem.

—L. R. Knost

May 2009

*Hannah is in this school year's last month of developmental preschool
at four years old, and Connor is two. Our fenced-in back yard has provided entertainment for both of them while I made dinner.*

*I set the table and call the kids in from outside. Connor is quick to
react, but Hannah is not. On the third call, I have her attention, and
her exaggerated high step over the door's track reveals her ongoing proprioception difficulties. I drain the spaghetti and dish it and the sauce
onto our plates. Hannah's pasta needs to be cut up extra-fine.*

*Now I'm ready to help the kids wash their hands. Connor is al-
ready at the table, so I just pick him up and we head to the hallway
restroom. I quickly wash Connor's hands and call for Hannah. No
response. "Hannah!" Clearly, she is not listening to me. I drop off Connor in the kitchen and head off to find her. Not in the family room,
not in the makeshift playroom, formal living room, or dining room.*

Ugh! Upstairs. Not in her bedroom, not in Connor's bedroom, nor in our bedroom or bathroom. I look around the guest bedroom, but no Hannah.

Where is she? Now I scream her name. "Hannah!" I know she couldn't have opened the patio screen door—she lacks the strength. As I descend the steps, I can see outside and remember: I had opened the front door. All she had to do was press the handle on the storm door. I run into the front yard. I don't want to alert the neighbors yet, but she's not there—not in the driveway, not in the street. I must have missed her in the house. *I know it's ridiculous, but I look under couch cushions, in the coat closet, and in the laundry room. Too much time has passed. I can't deny it anymore. She's gone! She went out the front door and is either wandering our neighborhood or someone has picked her up! This can't be happening!*

I run outside again, and the president of our homeowner's association is in his yard, which is next to ours. He always seems to be a calm guy with a methodical mind. He'll help me!

"Brian, Hannah is missing! Hannah is missing!" I plead as if he has the ability to instantly locate my girl. He goes into his house, rallies his family, and they set out in all directions to search our neighborhood. Meanwhile, my friend and classroom aide, Ed, pulls into our driveway with his wife. They also live in the neighborhood and can tell I've pushed the panic button. Their eyes have no answers.

I go into the house and call my husband. Thank goodness the call goes right through to his office. He assures me he'll come home immediately. I call my best friend, Lori, who lives only minutes away. She answers right away and promises to be here as soon as she can.

I walk outside in a slow-motion blur. People have converged in my yard. There are more people combing our streets and sidewalks than I've ever seen outside their homes. Then, I see it—the police car. This is happening. This is real. She's gone. Why did I leave the front door open? Why does she wander? How could she have been here one minute and gone the next? Does someone have her? Has she reached the pond yet? No, there hasn't been time. I yell to have someone check.

While I walk back into the house, I know the police will want to talk to me. I try to recall what she's wearing. The house is quiet compared to the sounds of panic outside. I touch my chest and force myself to breathe. Connor has given up on dinner and is playing with his Lincoln Logs. I grab Hannah's picture off the mantel. Maybe the police will need this. *I can see into the playroom where Connor is building.*

Hannah pops up! She was hiding in a nook behind the toy box. "Mommy," *she says,* "Me no eat."

"What? You were behind the toy box all this time?" I rush over to grab her and hold her as tightly as I can. My friend, Lori, must have heard. She's on the couch with us. Hannah's on my lap and I'm sobbing. "I love you, honey, I love you, I love you." Then I pull her back and look her in the eyes. "We were so worried! Please don't do that again! Please come when Mommy calls!" I squeeze her against me even though I know she hates close contact and I rock back and forth, back and forth. "I love you, I love you, I love you . . ."

I finally catch my breath and feel the adrenaline slowing its frantic pulse through my body. I pull her away from me again so I can ask, "Why did you hide from us? Just because you didn't want to eat?"

No response. She stares at the back of the couch instead of making eye contact. I can't stop asking, "Couldn't you tell that I was worried? Didn't you know what you were doing was wrong?" Lori is rubbing my shoulders as I continue, "You can't do that to me again, Hannah! We were so afraid. We thought you were gone. Why? Why can't you understand me?"

The second stage of interventions (ages three to nine) continued to be challenging. As you can see from the flashback, feeding was no exception. We would soon learn that Hannah's feeding challenges weren't only a texture sensitivity issue but also an **interoception** challenge. A relatively unheard of sensory system, interoception is responsible for detecting internal regulation responses such as respiration, hunger, heart rate, and the need for elimination. Hence her ongoing struggles with eating and digestion.

Hannah was also growing older. I put pressure on myself to have her ready for kindergarten. Dr. Jed Baker coined a term that could have described me during this stage—a healthy neurotic. I was Hannah's dedicated, staunch case manager fighting desperately to find any avenue that would help her feel more comfortable in her own skin, including keeping her on track with school so she would be in the same grade as her peers. But the world was too intense for her brain. Did I possibly overdo it during this time? Yes. However, it was clear to me how great her deficits were and how much was required to give her every chance of emerging to her full potential. Would I do the same things if I had to do it all over again? Yes. And you can too!

This chapter recalls our struggles, missteps, and successes. See how, anchored by hope, we would never give up on our daughter and know that your interventions are not in vain. And over time, my concept of *normal* did change—which was comforting.

FACTS ABOUT AUTISM SPECTRUM DISORDER[11]

* ASD is a neurodevelopmental disorder that affects social communication and social interaction as well as behaviors, interests, and activities.
* It is common for ASD to co-occur with other developmental, psychiatric, neurologic, chromosomal, and/or genetic diagnoses.
* ASD affects individuals of all races, ethnicities, social classes, lifestyles, and educational backgrounds equally.
* ASD cannot be cured, but there are many treatment options that enable individuals with ASD to compensate for areas of challenge.
* Individuals with ASD may demonstrate attachment or affectionate behaviors to parents and/or caregivers; however, such attachment or affection may be on the individual's own terms or expressed in a manner that is different from what society would typically expect.
* Individuals with ASD often have individual strengths and weaknesses across academic and functional areas; however, a few individuals with ASD have savant abilities.

❖ ASD is more common in boys than girls with 1 in 54 boys being affected in comparison to 1 in 252 girls or approximately 5 boys to every 1 girl receiving an ASD diagnosis.

MISCONCEPTIONS ABOUT AUTISM SPECTRUM DISORDER[12]

People need the facts (see previous text box) about ASD or else they hold to and spread these misconceptions, making it harder for people with the diagnosis to get the help they need.

❖ Autism spectrum disorder is an emotional problem.
❖ Individuals can be affected by ASD or another disorder, but they cannot be affected by multiple disorders.
❖ ASD occurs more often in people with high incomes and higher levels of education.
❖ ASD can be cured.
❖ Individuals with ASD do not become attached or show affection to others.
❖ All children with ASD have savant abilities in specific areas.
❖ The occurrence of ASD is equal between boys and girls.

TIME FOR SCHOOL: PRESCHOOL EXPERIENCES

In February 2008 it was time to take a giant step—developmental preschool. This meant Hannah would get picked up by a school bus in the morning at daycare, receive OT, PT, and ST at one of our district's elementary schools, get life skills instruction from a trained special education teacher to learn routines like eating and toilet training, and utilize tools such as a visual picture schedule, a Time Timer, and a weighted sensory vest. Professionals would test Hannah's IQ and perform evaluations to see if she qualified for each of the therapies, and I would need to complete more behavioral and sensory profiles. My husband and I attended the state's general transition meeting, which happened to be hosted by our school district. We learned that our school district had received favorable referrals from medical professionals because of its admirable special education programs. This insight provided comfort and confirmed that our move was warranted—Hannah was where she needed to be. The administrators provided a thorough description of the program, and my husband and I took detailed notes. Our next step was to meet with the intake coordinator in our home.

INTAKE PROCESS—INITIAL STEPS

The intake coordinator and her husband had worked in our district for quite some time. Although I didn't personally know her, she made me feel comfortable and I sensed mutual respect between us. I could tell that she knew her job well and was vested in making a difference in Hannah's life. When you find authentic treasures in a person like this, seize the opportunity to take advantage of their skill sets. She was one of the few professionals I wouldn't need to pay or convince to help my daughter make great strides. Special needs educators have made a choice to work with our population of children for a reason. Don't forget that! As parents, we didn't have a choice whether to have a special needs child or not, but these professionals could have opted for a different field and yet chose to dedicate themselves to helping children like ours succeed. The intake coordinator made me feel nurtured from the very beginning.

The intake coordinator had Hannah's First Steps paperwork and discussed how the developmental preschool's services compared with First Steps. She explained the evaluation process, and we set a date. "I know you believe Hannah has autism," she said, "but we really need a diagnosis if you want to include that in her IEP." The diagnosis would allow Hannah services from the system's autism consultant. She then discussed the difference between an educational and medical diagnosis of autism. I sighed and handed over Hannah's two summative medical diagnoses of autism and added that Hannah's neurologist and developmental pediatrician could provide additional summative evaluations if needed.

When those papers left my hands, I felt I had done my job. I had already taken the necessary steps to get Hannah into the program best suited to her needs. Be proactive and do everything possible to expedite services.

Just before the meeting ended, the intake coordinator handed us *the blue folder.*

A NEW REALITY

That dreadful blue folder. It sat on our dining room table for two whole weeks without being touched. We'd already made the appointment for our evaluation, so I knew it could sit for a while. I didn't take one peek at its contents—an unprecedented, uncharacteristic choice on my part. No matter the news, I had always acted immediately on anything Hannah needed to make meaningful gains. Not this time. I wanted to throw it away, burn it, and I sure as hell knew it didn't belong on my table or in my possession.

When she qualified, that *blue folder* would officially enroll Hannah in our school system's special education program. My daughter would be a special needs student. I knew this was the right next step for her, but what was so special about it? One of the two virtues I had respected the most, I felt my daughter would never be able to possess—intelligence. Kindness is the other virtue, and time will tell if she develops that as an individual and special needs student. Sounds horrible, doesn't it? I admit it. Knowledge is power, and I had an insatiable hunger for it and wanted all children—especially my own—to grow in knowledge and develop intelligence and communication skills.

I remember how I'd see children her age in large superstores, unsupervised and dirty, but walking and talking effortlessly—even running! The educator in me was glad they were developing despite what seemed to be less than stellar attention from their caregivers. The parent in me, though—the parent of a child with autism—struggled. How was this fair? Why were those parents rewarded with children who functioned normally and hit developmental stages effortlessly? Why was my daughter so behind, despite access to multiple therapies? After all this effort, why would she still be in a program for kids who could not function at the same level of these youngsters? Why the blue folder for Hannah and mainstreamed classes for the rest of the world? I knew this was judgmental and wrong, but I felt raw. This was my heart and mind, unfiltered. Envy, frustration, and devastation were real. I mourned, and my grief manifested as sadness, anxiety attacks, and hair loss. Negative emotions have the power to drain us of our strength.

It's normal to have these thoughts and feelings. Don't feel guilty—it means you're human. Deal with them in a way that feels healthy, but I urge you not to stay in that place or dwell on it. Acknowledge, and forgive yourself (and others) if that's what will free you and keep you from staying stuck. As parent advocates, we can't stay there. Our kids need us as attentive and positive as possible as we head into evaluation and testing.

EVALUATION AND TESTING

We dropped Hannah off to the evaluation team one afternoon, and she was done within two hours. The team reported that she had done a nice job and was well behaved. They would actually become Hannah's teachers and therapists if she qualified—which didn't take a professional to deduce. At this time, we also handed in the blue folder and set an appointment for her psychological testing.

The psychological testing was done at my school in the office's conference room. Hannah was restless at first, so the evaluator allowed me to stay for a while. The school psychologist used a variety of methods to engage Hannah—none worked. Hannah was quiet and regulated, but mentally not there. Hannah could not perform any of the defined tasks. She offered no eye contact, no pointing, no making choices— nothing. No participation of any kind.

I felt another jolt. This was my daughter—unable to respond or react to the most basic tasks and interaction. I left the room agitated, pacing the hallway, thinking, worried, wondering what was next— what was to become of my daughter? The psychologist paged me after a short time. Hannah's IQ did not measure. In other words, Hannah didn't have the cognitive ability to even take the test that would measure her intelligence.

Suffering on top of suffering. On the drive home, I glanced at her when we stopped at lights. *Are those tests right? Is there truly not any measurable intelligence in my daughter? Nothing at all?*

FIRST CONFERENCE

We met in early January 2008 for Hannah's first official case conference. Everyone commented that stadium seating should have been assembled. As a parent and a teacher, I recommend going into the annual case reviews with the mindset that the schools and teachers have your child's best interest at heart. I share more on this in chapter 10. I specifically asked all of Hannah's therapists from First Steps to attend. They could help us make sense of the evaluation team's interdisciplinary report. They also knew what worked and didn't work for Hannah. I basically wanted them to consult with Hannah's new team to develop a plan (an IEP) that would work best. This is a bold move, as schools don't suggest this. You'll have to be proactive and confident, but I'm glad I did and I'm glad they all came. Resolve to be the advocate and make those phone calls to ensure your child gets an accurate review.

As a teacher, I had attended a multitude of case conferences to discuss students' needs and IEPs, but this was different. This was *my* child. Being on the other side of the table felt foreign and uncomfortable. After introductions and the obligatory offer of procedural safeguards (procedural safeguards spell out what the school can and can't do when evaluating and providing special education and related services to your child), my husband and I asked to read a letter composed just for Hannah's new team. I wrote the two-page letter but insisted that my husband read it, as his demeanor is powerful, yet sincere. The letter explained the tumultuous storm of our past year and a half. We discussed Dr. Pappas's devastating prognosis that Hannah would never leave a Life Skills classroom. That's when our school psychologist, who has a son with autism, left the room. I felt my stomach lurch—I was only thinking about our own family and didn't realize our words might affect another family struggling through the same processes.

We told the committee about Hannah's progress with the thera-pists, but also shared the areas of greatest concern. The letter explained how Hannah lost skills if not repeated daily. We described her failure to thrive. My husband paused several times to clear his throat, gather his emotions, and compose himself. We explained how frustrating it was to be educators and not be able to teach our own daughter. We shared the puzzle analogy and explained the evident missing pieces in Hannah's receptive and expressive language—how we longed to start talking with her and have her understand our words and one day understand hers. We made sure they understood her inability to read facial expressions and nonverbal clues as well as her sensory processing disorder and its effect on her not being able to experi-ence the world. We implored them to help find the missing pieces and put them back together again. Though the puzzle analogy may sound cliché to those familiar with the world of autism, it was fresh and ap-plicable to us. Each person heard our hearts—I looked up from the letter and saw people wiping away tears. We had humbled ourselves in front of the fifteen people all gathered in a conference room de-signed for ten—even more, we had ripped out our hearts, set them on a plate, and asked everyone to treat them as tenderly as if they were their own.

Everyone around the table on the evaluation team said that Han-nah did qualify for the maximum amount of time on their service. This didn't surprise me. The autism consultant discussed what she could offer Hannah with personalized stories, PECS cards, video modeling, social pragmatic skills, and available resources for behav-ior management. The school psychologist returned to the room and shared the testing she had done with Hannah. Cognitively, Hannah's aptitude was assumed to be well below the average standard—as she was unable to take the IQ test. The other behaviors the testing re-vealed were just as concerning and still linger as possible for Hannah to manifest today. The tests declared that Hannah was fearful, at risk for anxiety and depression, exhibiting behaviors suggesting obses-sive-compulsive disorder, and at risk for **somatization disorder**. How do you swallow that? Such somber words, and I had no desire at the time to even ask what in the world somatization disorder was. Your mind can't wrap itself around the words uttered by another about your child. You stop breathing, your head gets fuzzy, and tears refuse to be summoned—shock sets in. My poor baby. Just a preschooler, and we'd heard nothing but dire outcomes. I needed to go home, pull the covers over my head, and just be.

NO TIME TO PROBE BIG QUESTIONS—TIME TO GET PRACTICAL

At that time, in that moment, I wanted a cure. I wanted answers. What made Hannah like this? What caused her autism? I didn't have time to dig into it, and I knew there probably wasn't a cure, but boy did I want one. For now, I had to move on. You'll have to move on as well. Time to get on the bus . . .

MOCK BUS RIDE

Hannah and I were allowed a mock bus ride prior to her first day of school. Truth be told, it was more for me than Hannah. My husband and I were wary. Who wants to put their three-year-old on a bus? Hannah and I were able to meet her driver and bus aide. The aide helped her tackle the steps, removed her backpack, buckled her in her seat, and around the neighborhood we went!

The mock bus ride went better than I had anticipated. When facing times of uncertainty about your child's well-being, don't be afraid to suggest a mock bus ride or even a classroom observation. Schools and teachers are usually amenable, and it will do wonders for your peace of mind as a parent.

PRESCHOOL BEGINS

On her first day of school, anticipation was tough for all of the adults at the bus stop—but not Hannah. I still remember that cold rainy day with Hannah in her stretchy, comfortable outfit with her monogrammed backpack in tow. Her teacher had created a personalized story introducing the daily routine, faces, and environment. Most moms have two and a half more years before facing this moment, so it was bittersweet to let go this early. Cameras flashed while camcorders documented this monumental day in my daughter's education. After the bus took off, my husband followed it to school. And he has done so every first day of school for both of our children.

Hannah attended the preschool every weekday morning through May. Every day, the school staff worked on the goals listed in her IEP. Communication was key to accelerating progress. A notebook traveled from home to school daily. I have kept them all. Teachers and therapists were expected to document attempted tasks with challenges and send instructions home for how to reinforce the skills. We would return the notebook with comments on how she fared in the home environment. Before the school year ended, the committee was quick to amend Hannah's IEP, enabling her to take advantage of the extended school year option of two weeks. The committee was concerned that too much time away from school might cause a regression of skills. For Hannah we had to teach, reteach, teach, reteach and then continually review for her to retain the skill.

PRESCHOOL AND MORE PRESCHOOL

In the fall I decided to bump up the rigor a notch. My friend, Lori, sat on the board of her church's preschool (Play-N-Share), which was right across the street from where we taught. Three-year-olds attended two days a week in the afternoons. What if Hannah attended developmental preschool every morning and Play-N-Share on Monday and Wednesday afternoons? Thank goodness for our daycare. They agreed to provide transportation to and from Play-N-Share. We asked the director if she would take Hannah—would she accept into the program a child with autism? Would she say no? I walked into her office clutching my folder packed with notes, prepared to advocate for Hannah in hopes of convincing her to say yes. We met eyes, and I realized I'd taught her daughter in school. She remembered me. Always nice to know someone.

Before entering her office, I'd decided to be nonchalant about Hannah's challenges. Well, that didn't last long. I don't believe I've ever been nonchalant about a thing in my life. All of a sudden, it all spewed out—the autism, its challenges, and my desire for Hannah to be mainstreamed with typical kids her age so she could experience some type of normalcy. Maybe it was me that needed the normalcy? The director didn't even blink an eye. No concerned look or uncertainty. I was perplexed.

"Tell me more about Hannah," she said. I heard nothing in her voice that implied she would deny Hannah's admission. I spilled out every detail and she listened to every word. The director reassured me Hannah would be welcome in the program and informed me about the preschool's best in-house resource—a teacher who also had a child on the spectrum.

HANNAH STARTS TO EMERGE

That school year was busy. Hannah made some small gains that renewed our hope, but challenges remained. I was still driving her to weekly feeding therapy. We also had our private OT come once a week. My school system was also kind enough to check in with Hannah at Play-N-Share and give her teachers any advice they might need.

Hannah slowly began to use her words (expressive language). By age three and a half, she had a ten-word vocabulary, then entered a stage when she spoke a lot of gibberish—an attempt to communicate. Shortly after this time, Hannah started using **echolalia** and could recite a lot of the lines to her favorite shows, including *Dora the Explorer*. Children with autism use echolalia because they long to speak, but aren't able to put the words together. I was fortunate enough to hear Dr. Barry Prizant, author of *Uniquely Human*, speak in 2017 at the Autism Society of America's national conference in Milwaukee, Wisconsin. Dr. Prizant said that he believes that echolalia is communicative. His book states the anecdotal evidence for his belief. Did Hannah really understand the words, or was she just memorizing them and repeating them back? I decided it was the latter due to her poor receptive and expressive language ability. However, she was still trying to communicate.

To augment the therapist's efforts, I reinforced what they taught her and integrated my own ideas. To help Hannah's receptive language and motor planning, for example, I started to ask Hannah questions in a slow manner, provide wait time, answer them for her, and then have her repeat the answer. This trained her to return expressive language. If I had to do this the rest of her life to allow her to function at a higher level, then I decided that's what I'd do. I became Hannah's voice because she had my heart. She would still flap to modulate herself, but I didn't mind. Hannah flapped because she wanted so badly to communicate. She didn't choose to be silent; her brain's synapses just weren't firing to make the connections as quickly as they needed to.

Her receptive language slowly started to improve, and she understood some of what we were saying. She continued to use her voice for counting, saying colors, and noticing shapes and patterns in our environment. She didn't have to discern meaning from numbers, colors, or shapes, so the rote memorization made language acquisition easier for her. We used flashcards with words to help her understand that letters make words and words make sentences. Hannah grew obsessed with the cards and started memorizing the words. Now, instead of using the PECS cards for her needs, she was learning, "I want . . ."

She was now four and slowly accomplished potty training and walking down steps. Believe it or not, what motivated Hannah to finally brave walking down the steps was the certainty that she would be able to count them, and there would always be a complete seventeen in our home. I decided with relief—and perhaps the beginning of hope, even joy—that *a little bit of progress* is autism's true definition.

END-OF-YEAR REVIEW

At Hannah's end-of-the-year case conference, the school system offered an unbelievable opportunity that validated Hannah's hard work. They proposed to "bus" Hannah to a well-known academic preschool (Light and Life) in our town to transition Hannah the following year to a regular kindergarten. Shocked—and secretly thrilled—I had been ready to suggest that Hannah spend the coming year and an extra year in developmental preschool before even attempting kindergarten.

The transition coordinator would meet with the preschool's director and Hannah's teacher to discuss modifications and accommodations, and she would also periodically observe Hannah and give feedback. Our school system's autism consultant would also be videoing Hannah several times during the year to document successes as well as challenges. Best yet, state-allotted preschool funding paid the tuition. I couldn't believe it! The committee was suggesting a rigorous, typical preschool environment for Hannah. She would be bused back to the elementary school on Mondays, Wednesdays, and Fridays for her therapies. The school system provided all of the transportation to and from daycare. Fortunately, this wasn't something I had to fight for or understand every detail of special needs law to request. The school system informed me of this opportunity. Expect the same courtesy from your school system.

TIME FOR SCHOOL: MAINSTREAM PRESCHOOL

It was a little funny. Parents would arrive in cars to drop off their children, and Hannah would arrive in a big yellow school bus with only one other child on board. The bus aide would even accompany both of them in and out. Obviously, Hannah was oblivious to the outside world and had no idea she was getting there any differently than anyone else. I was terrified that Hannah would still not be able to attend regular kindergarten the following year, so to continue maximizing her progress, Hannah continued to also go to Play-N-Share on Tuesday and Thursday afternoons.

PRESCHOOL ORGANIZATION

Planning for school was the hardest part. Basically, there were three different schools with different schedules, meals and snack times, folders, letters of the week, teachers, themes, and programs. We stopped private OT at this time. In the beginning Hannah struggled each morning because she didn't know what to expect for her day. We created a simple picture schedule using PECS cards. This lowered her anxiety levels.

A WAY TO INTERACT WITH OTHERS

Hannah's eye contact really improved during this year, but she still wasn't interacting with her peers. Her teacher at Light and Life had a brilliant idea. As a result of our work with memorizing sight words, her love for our alone time reading picture books, and her time on starfall. com (a free children's reading tutorial website), Hannah had learned to actually read children's books. The teacher would place Hannah in a rocking chair in front of her peers. Hannah would read children's picture books to them. Her reading fluency was now off the charts. Later I would learn that this ability is referred to as **hyperlexia**—a syndrome characterized by a child's precocious ability to read, combined with difficulty in understanding and using verbal language and problems with social interactions. So, yes, Hannah learned to read before learning how to spontaneously generate sentences on her own.

PRESCHOOL GRADUATION TIMES THREE

In May 2010 Hannah officially graduated from three preschools. I could not have been prouder. At Play-N-Share's graduation, students had to announce future career aspirations. I was nervous, but the teachers had prepped Hannah. They called her name. She went to the microphone wearing her semi-formal royal blue and fuchsia dress, looked at the audience, threw her hands up in the air, and said very slowly—while wearing the biggest grin I'd ever witnessed from my daughter: "I want to be everything!" I believe she was truly happy. Hannah was five, and she didn't show "happy" that often. This. This moment was worth all those hours of therapy, all those complicated schedules, all those worries and fears. For this moment in time, Hannah was expressing something beautiful, unique, and utterly true. She was emerging.

TIME FOR ELEMENTARY SCHOOL

Hannah was being mainstreamed into a general education kindergarten class. When meeting at the end of the year for her case conference, the staff discussed Hannah's kindergarten round-up scores. This pre-assessment is administered to every incoming kindergarten student. The committee suggested that Hannah spend reading class in a first grade classroom. First grade! This, the girl who didn't score on an IQ test two years prior, now reading a grade level up! I was so proud of her and wished she could feel it, too. Phonics would be a waste of her time since she had already learned to read. For socialization, I wish I would have kept her with the same kids all day, but in the long run, it was fine.

After Hannah's first day of kindergarten, I anxiously awaited at daycare for her bus to arrive. The new bus driver and aide had trouble finding Hannah's drop-off, and the driver couldn't contact the transportation center. Of course Hannah was not able to help the driver with the location. Hannah returned to daycare forty-five minutes later than scheduled. Sobbing, I had called her patient principal, who stayed on the phone with me until Hannah's safe return.

As her aide helped her off the bus, I saw that her new shirt was covered with chocolate milk. She doesn't even drink chocolate milk, so I checked her communication log and apparently she had tried to drink from the carton because she was not able to ask for a straw—let alone white milk. Hannah, unable to find the right words, string them together, and articulate them, while struggling to sense where her body was in space, had poured the chocolate milk all over herself. And she was limping! She wasn't able to explain what had happened. At Back-to-School Night that evening I inquired. Hannah had attempted the monkey bars for the first time ever in her life, but lacked the needed upper body strength. She'd fallen, hard. My husband and I took her to the orthopedist the next morning (our second day of school as well) because she was still limping. Sure enough, our little girl had broken a small bone in her foot. The doctor couldn't believe her pain tolerance. Instead of placing a cast, due to her overtaxed sensory system, Hannah was able to heal in a medical walking boot so small, it looked like it was made for her American Girl doll. The next day, her special education Teacher of Record made a personalized story about what equipment she could and could not access.

During times like this, we must learn to have patience with the school system and school. There's so much to remember about each child, and Hannah's class had thirty students. As a teacher, I know that it takes time to understand each child's specific needs. No parent or teacher can plan that the "unexpected" could happen. Hannah's Individualized Education Plan didn't say she was not allowed to play on the monkey bars or required a straw to drink milk, nor can anyone plan a last minute bus driver change. Be careful of the stress that can be unintentionally applied to the education system. That's not to recommend passivity or excuse patterns of negligence—if the school did nothing to correct the first day blunders, that would be different—but trust the school system to act in the student's best interest. Hannah's always has.

Hannah learned that year to say, "Hi! My name is Hannah. Want to play?" It sounded scripted, awkward, but before long, it became more fluid. Scripting can be a powerful tool in preparing your child for social interactions. Then, over time, we realized Hannah also completely stopped flapping in direct correlation with her speech development. When she began to find her voice, her agitation eased up. Just as I always suspected, the flapping was about communication. My little girl had tons to say, but couldn't articulate the words. During Hannah's kindergarten year, a friend of mine who taught fourth grade formed "Book Buddies" with Hannah's class. The fourth graders even performed a play together with the kindergarteners, and Hannah had a few lines as a princess! I thanked my friend and Hannah's teacher for the extra effort that helped my daughter shine—look for ways to do that in your situation, as well. They need to know how important their programs and ideas are for the child and to the family.

Hannah was gradually dismissed from physical and speech therapy services throughout first and second grades. She remained on consultation services only for occupational therapy. The autism and behavioral consultants would lead discussions centered around building and maintaining friendships, and communicating emotions. Hannah also had a room of respite if needed—the guidance counselor's office, which was stocked with sensory toys and books—and her teachers and I stopped journaling back and forth. Hannah continued to transition to an advanced grade for reading class. The school discussed the option of grade-skipping with us, but emotionally she was years behind her peers. I knew this decision should not be made on intellect alone. Hannah's language continued to materialize, and she was beginning to interact more with people at least on a surface level—I didn't want to thrust her into more advanced communication when she was gaining ground with peers.

After these two years, Hannah was also able to ride a regular school bus. I found comfort knowing that her brother, a mere kindergartner himself, would be on the same bus. Even though Hannah's behavior, interactions, and eating were all still challenges, her deficits were beginning to not be so glaring. She didn't have groups of friends, but she had one good friend. During these years she would continually tell me that I was her angel's wings. While interventions began to level off and she progressed at a steady pace, our pace of life started to seem slower, sustainable, and more normal than it had ever been.

At the end of her second grade year, Hannah tested into our school system's High Ability Program. She was then labeled by her neurologist with Asperger's syndrome. Asperger's syndrome does fall within the realm of autism, but individuals are characterized by higher than average intellectual capabilities. Subsequently, the latest DSM-5 removed the label of Asperger's syndrome to categorize it, once again, as solely autism.

Given Hannah's new placement, she continued to thrive academically in her High Ability cohort for third and fourth grade. Being with the same peers all day for two years was comforting to her. They understood and accepted her, though her teachers reported that she had trouble working in groups and struggled to see others' point of view. That came as no surprise to me. Hannah still has trouble giving others permission to have a point of view. She also had difficulty with constructive criticism. She didn't understand that others were trying to be helpful and the input was directed to help her, not discourage her.

Hannah wanted friendships so badly, but social conventions continued to baffle her. She would make a friend and cling so tightly emotionally she would scare them off. Hannah also didn't understand that peers don't like to be publicly corrected. This certainly didn't help build friendships. Her closest of friends were her toys, her cat, and her books.

By fourth grade, she wasn't receiving any services from the school system besides occasional consultation with the autism consultant and accommodations or modifications in the classroom. During these years, she earned second place in our county's oratorical contest and was chosen to represent her school in Math Bowl. Her conceptual understanding of math enabled her to know more than the isolated facts and methodology. She was able to see mathematical ideas in her head and transfer those to new situations—which was relaxing for her. Math was the language she understood best. Abstract problems were met conceptually and logically in her mind.

And she had found a place on the stage! When time for the fourth grade drama rolled around, she earned a lead as Mrs. Potts in *Beauty and the Beast.* Due to her involvement in the oratorical contest and *Beauty and the Beast,* she became a quick study on nonverbal communication and facial expressions. That year she also received the award for Art Student of the Year. Happiness!

ADDITIONAL THERAPIES

Hannah participated in two additional therapies during the grade-school years: equine-assisted therapy and aquatic therapy. I chose therapies based on what I thought would work for Hannah within our financial resources—not necessarily therapies that were convenient for me.

EQUINE-ASSISTED THERAPY

Another parent recommended equine-assisted therapy to help with Hannah's poor upper body strength and lack of focus. Hannah's unabashed love for nature and animals convinced me to pursue it. A horse named Magic and a therapist named Molly created another environment that met Hannah in her world and pulled her into ours. This therapy actually stretched me. The heat, smell, thousands of flies, clouds of dust—not to mention the wandering goats, llamas, cats, and chickens—left me longing for Purell and a bubble bath. But it wasn't about me. Magic and Molly were building bridges from Hannah to us while increasing her focus and strength—for that I'll shoo away a thousand flies, or a million!

AQUATIC THERAPY

During Hannah's time in developmental preschool, our school system hosted an Autism Fair. I was surprised to see our school's physical education lifeguard, Katinka, at the fair. "I've always loved teaching kids with autism to swim!" She explained how comforting water pressure is to kids, as it allows body awareness as the water pressure is distributed equally. "Water has a calming effect on these kids and a lot of time I'll see them talk more, stim less, and even maintain eye contact. Hannah should try it!" We signed her up on the spot, and Hannah took to it like, well, a fish to water. Hannah interacted with Katinka, and the water provided an ideal medium for Hannah to thrive. Hannah was prone to meltdowns triggered by environmental factors that were unidentifiable at times, but after a session with Katinka, Hannah was able to control her emotions and anxiety. She always understood and followed Katinka's instructions in the water without delay. This therapy complicated our schedule, added significant cost to our budget, and increased bath and laundry time—and it stripped Hannah's hair of healthy natural oils. But it was all worth it. Every afternoon Hannah emerged from that pool, I could see her emerging just a little bit more from the limits we thought autism had placed on her.

ACTIVITIES

As you can see, I don't want to miss out on any chance of seeing my daughter arrive at her full potential, so in addition to the therapies and school events, I signed up Hannah for other activities that I hoped would be fun and provide additional benefits.

BALLET

Hannah loved classical music, so I signed her up for ballet for two years because I thought it would be a pleasant connection with the music while improving her gross motor movement. Other kids in the class didn't understand that Hannah had autism and would often help her by dragging her little arm on the dance floor to the spot where she was supposed to be. Thankfully, Hannah didn't respond with violent meltdowns from being touched. The kids were accepting, and the moms were impressed that Hannah was picking up and reading children's books in the waiting room. This made me proud—they weren't pitying her deficits, but praising her talents! The biggest benefit Hannah derived from ballet was not only the fact that her gross motor skills became more fluid, but Hannah had to actually "watch" the teacher in the front of the studio and mimic her movements. That was an association that couldn't be missed.

GYMNASTICS

When equine-assisted therapy and ballet were finished, I enrolled Hannah in gymnastics to continue improving her upper body strength. I had never realized the role upper body strength plays in our daily lives until Hannah lacked it. Closing a car door, opening a store door, fastening a seat belt, picking up a back pack, and accessing playground equipment all required more strength than she had. With gymnastics, she gained dramatic strength and while she wasn't operating at a competitive level, she was strong. I'd watch her swing on the uneven bars and feel my heart soar.

BASKETBALL

A lot of kids in our state play basketball, so it seemed right to sign up Hannah for a basketball club at our local YMCA. This sport requires coordination and the capacity to understand the team concept as well as lots of rules.

It proved too much for my girl at first. Fortunately, the kids were so young, the officials were lenient. One time Hannah got the ball, carried—without dribbling—the ball all of the way to her team's basket, and shot. Lacking upper body strength to heave the ball to the rim, she missed. She was devastated. The other kids retrieved the ball and continued play while Hannah stood in place without moving, chest heaving with impending wails or screams—who knows what.

The coach saw her and stopped the game. He spoke to the officials, and they handed Hannah the ball. She ran off the court with the ball, up the bleachers, and right into my lap. I knew how Hannah processed the world most comfortably—through concrete, mathematical ideas. So I pointed to the clock and said, "Hannah, you have forty-five seconds to get this sphere into that circle." She was hugging the ball. I patted it and pointed to the basket. "That circle's diameter is bigger than the ball's diameter, so you can do this. Stand closer to the circle. See the square behind the circle?" She nodded. Her meltdown had calmed. I continued, "Maybe you can bounce this sphere off that square into the circle. What do you think?" She nodded again, slowly, then walked down the bleachers and shot. Missed. Shot again. Missed. The coach went out onto the floor, put Hannah onto his shoulders, and told her to shoot the ball again. She made the shot! The bleachers exploded with cheers and applause. And that was the end of my girl's career with basketball. Not all of our efforts will prove to be fruitful, but we learn something from every one of them.

BEHAVIORS

Children with autism need behaviors treated—not the diagnosis itself. Every behavior has an antecedent, or trigger. Hannah had many challenging behaviors during this stage that we addressed primarily with medication and rules conveyed with precise language.

MEDICATION

Hannah became obsessed with walking the perimeter of rooms, not stepping on lines, pushing buttons, and picking her nails. All of these were nonfunctional rituals. I had remembered in the movie, *Rain Man*, Dustin Hoffman's character with autism had fixated on pushing buttons too!

When her methodical preferences weren't met, she'd collapse on the ground, kicking and screaming. These meltdowns began impacting the rest of the family so that we could barely function. We decided it was time to ask her doctor to prescribe the minimum amount of medication to help her behaviors. He prescribed liquid Paxil.

We were so afraid that instead of changing the behaviors we would only mask the problems, but if these behaviors became ingrained, they might be even harder to extinguish. So, at age four, that's what we did. Before the medication, she could not stop the downward spiral to the kicking and screaming. Within two months of a low dose of doctor-prescribed medication, she could actually stop the meltdown just as it was beginning and we could continue with dinner, go to the event we were heading to, or make it to the car without any resistance. Don't feel like a failure if you, too, have to resort to medication to help your child process the world. Their challenges are sometimes out of our control.

PRECISION AND RULES

There are several situations in which Hannah has displayed unique differences. She always needed to know immediately where certain items and objects were located. When she was younger, it was mainly toys. I kept the kids' toys organized so I could find the right toy Hannah wanted before a meltdown.

She never wanted to participate in any of her schools' pajama days. In Hannah's words, "Pajamas are only to be worn at bedtime. Why would anyone wear them to school?"

She also established a strict bedtime regimen that she was finally able to abandon. We always had to read the same book, *You Are My I Love You*. The book had a hidden animal on each page, and Hannah always had to find it. I then needed to sing "You Are My Sunshine," and then "I love yous" were exchanged and a quick kiss. If I deviated from the script, she would insist on starting all over.

She never understood the importance of staying quiet during church, so we went a few years with meager attendance.

Being first in line was critical—so much so that she would rather leave an amusement park and ruin a trip rather than stand in line or board a ride after her brother. I offer solutions in chapter 8.

AFFINITIES

I always watched for Hannah's interests and affinities, and in these years she grew obsessed with cats, trains, astronomy, and specific series of books. Without attention to these topics, her face appeared vacant, so I jumped right into those proclivities with her. It's important that our children find motivation to explore their passions through those who love them. Showing your child that you care about his passion is the most powerful catalyst in the world.

Don't discount intense interests. They are your ticket for admission into your child's world. Temple Grandin's intense interest is animal behavior. Owen Suskind's intense interest is Disney films. Author of *Life, Animated*, Owen's father Ron Suskind said that parents are essentially codebreakers—cracking the code of our children's worlds in order for communication to take place. Once in their world, we gain their attention and use those affinities with a little wiggle room to bring new experiences into their lives.[13]

That's exactly what happened with Hannah. I knew every Thomas the Train engine in the set. We had astronomy flashcards, mobiles, books, an orbiting model of the solar system, and she had her own telescope. You may worry you're reinforcing the perseveration by focusing attention toward it. I encourage you to let that go, because those special interests are going to unlock possibilities of social interaction that will benefit your child's future. Use whatever it takes to get inside your child's world.

FINANCES AND PAPERWORK

Healthcare cost over a lifetime for an individual with autism or an intellectual challenge is 2.4 million dollars. Many have told me that state programs, like First Steps, are free. That wasn't our experience. Both of our salaries put us over the income threshold and a copay was required. Each appointment wasn't very expensive, but Hannah had four appointments a week, which added up over a year and a half. Needless to say, they were worth every penny. Autism does reset your priorities and your budget whether you like it or not.

There is a colossal amount of paperwork involved, along with phone calls and going back and forth with professionals and programs. For example, First Steps said that they accept insurance, but they had no one whose job was to bill insurance. Also, trying to figure out how to bill insurance for a private provider felt like a part-time job. Keeping track of the bills from weekly therapies was a must, then bills would need to be checked for accuracy to make sure insurance had paid first and we were only charged the residual. Even so, many of Hannah's services weren't covered by insurance. If I underestimated the importance of staying on top of the finances and paying on time, costs would have added up and further complicated our already complex lives. I suggest the use of an accordion folder to organize the financial statements from each of your providers. Keep a log on the front dating your correspondence and subject matter.

At this time, I also felt the looming need to establish a supplemental (special) needs trust every time I attended a workshop where financial advisors were present. Many parents don't realize that should anything happen to us, inheritance may cause many problems for our child with special needs. Under current federal law, any inheritance of more than two thousand dollars disqualifies individuals with disabilities from most federal needs-based assistance. Benefits from state public assistance programs may also be affected. A supplemental (special) needs trust offers a means of protecting your chid's eligibility for these benefits, while addressing the ongoing care and needs of your child with special needs.

I remember the time Hannah's speech therapist and I met to tour a full-time ABA facility. After touring the facility and observing its practices, we met with its director. I asked to see a price sheet on services offered. They looked surprised I would ask such a question. Apparently, they didn't believe it should be a factor to parents. They handed me the detailed schedule with astronomical prices. Shocked, I saw no way an assistant principal and a teacher could afford these services without declaring bankruptcy. I asked the director how families do it? He said, "Do you have a home? Do you have a vehicle? Wouldn't you give up everything to save Hannah?"

We had to apply for Hannah to be added to the autism waiver list for Medicaid. The wait could be long—up to ten years. We didn't know how Hannah's future would unfold, but we knew that applying would be a smart decision to gain resources and support to help cover a lifetime of services. The autism waiver from Medicaid would help to cover therapy appointments, respite services, and behavioral management. Hannah was granted the waiver eight years later. We currently only use the waiver for a behavioral management specialist and potential grants for ongoing autism education.

A CRYSTAL BALL

At this time in our lives, I craved a crystal ball to see into Hannah's future. What level of independence would the crystal ball reveal? Eventually I came to believe that whatever level of independence

Hannah attains will be a victory for my little girl. That beautiful acceptance was only possible over time. And believe me, acceptance doesn't mean giving up. When I heard Ron Suskind speak in New Orleans at the Autism Society of America's national conference in 2016, he asked, "Who decides what a meaningful life is anyway?" Enough said.

As parents, the second stage of interventions (ages three to nine) are the busiest time of our lives; however, the gains our children make during this time make it all worth it. Interventions are painful for us to watch and uncomfortable for our kids. I'll be honest, I'm still angry that our family was denied a typical toddlerhood for Hannah. Hannah's interventions drove our schedule.

You know what? She doesn't remember any of it—I do, but she doesn't. That makes it easier. Thankfully, even though our children are on the spectrum, they are resilient, brave, and strong. Be proud of their gains.

⚬⚬ **Wisdom from the Round Table** ⚬⚬

Lori R.: Cameron has a strict routine of going to bed and waking. He sets his alarm to go to bed at 9:30—not 9:29 or 9:31. He has to go by *his* watch and only hugs me. He gets out of bed at 7:30 on the dot—even if he has been awake for hours.

Jen: Noah has set his own rigid schedule. *Price is Right* is at 4:00. *Wheel of Fortune* while walking on the treadmill is at 7:00. Shower at 8:00. Deodorant at 9:30.

Lori V.: I can honestly say that it would be easy to become borderline obsessive about autism. In one year I counted 256 emails to Byron's teachers related to his autism. I became a parent advocate and quit a white-collar job in the pharmaceutical industry. My husband and I later divorced. With the economy being down and having been away from my career for more than five years, I had to take a minimum wage job at a local fast food establishment in order to try to support my family.

Susan: Those firsts that Bruce and I had to miss. First time we realized Tyler wouldn't be in a regular class, Tyler was never able to play on a basketball team, he wasn't able to get his driver's license, he never got to take a girl to prom. His sister and I are glad that he doesn't realize everything he's missing. The sponge gets full, and I cry and cry. Then, I'm fine. The cycle continually repeats itself.

Karen: We have always sought out great people and supports for both of our boys; however, I still continually beat myself up as a mother—never knowing if I've done enough.

Sarah: We refuse to let Mitchell's autism define his ability to succeed in school. I will not let him be held back, discriminated against, or left out due to Asperger's syndrome. I will not allow the barriers of his social abilities be ones he cannot climb.

CHAPTER EIGHT

holidays and vacations

Autism: Where the "randomness of life" collides and clashes with an individual's need for sameness.

—Ezra Taft Benson

December 2012

Hannah has her second grade Christmas program tonight. I shouldn't have put off finding her a special dress, but I did, and now it's an hour before the program. Time's up. It wasn't procrastination; it was the money. There simply isn't any extra now that my husband and I are going through a divorce. I never wanted my children to "want" for anything, but if I'm honest, I'm the only one who cares about the dress, not Hannah. As I pull last year's Christmas sweater dress over her head, I see that it's a little short—too much for my conservative dress values. I grab the sides of her dress and pull down with all of my might. It worked! I do the same to the front and the back. I'll dig up khaki shorts for her to wear underneath, just in case. She'll be up in the risers anyway.

Hannah's music teacher informed me last week via email that Hannah would be singing a small solo. Hannah continues to be challenged with conveying information from school to home. I get most updates by chance from other parents. I got the news about this solo early enough to invite my family and friends, who plan on meeting us there. No matter how small the solo, I want Hannah's moment in the spotlight to be celebrated.

As we arrive, I drop Hannah off at the cafeteria, and Connor and I find a good place to record the performance in the bleachers. Friends and family begin to show up, and now I'm on edge. Any change of schedule to Hannah's day usually causes disorientation—she craves a simple routine. I cannot truly relax and enjoy my family and friends like others. There could be a meltdown any time; I have to be ready, vigilant. Bleachers are now completely filled.

All four classes file into the gymnasium and begin organizing themselves onto the risers. I see Hannah, but she isn't looking for me. The first three songs are sung by the entire choir, and the kids look as if they're having fun. Every parent seems to be recording these precious moments with camcorders and iPhones.

Now it's time for the finale. An image of the movie The Polar Express is projected onto the large screen. The choir teacher pulls two microphone stands from behind the projector screen and lowers their height. I hold my breath and watch as students part to make room for Hannah and another little boy coming down the risers to claim their microphones. Hannah coughs into her elbow and begins scanning the audience intently. She needs to find me. I stand for a few fast seconds to bring attention to myself, and she gives me our universal sign that she's okay: a simple thumbs-up. I take a breath and ask someone else to record this moment for me.

The music starts for "When Christmas Comes to Town." The little boy steps up to the microphone and sings the first two verses. Now, Hannah's turn. She grabs the microphone with both hands and looks at me. She articulates the words, and with emotion! Her voice, amplified, sounds like she's proud of what she is doing. I never knew my daughter could sing! Hannah rocks this!

After her two verses, the music teacher hands both soloists a small bell. Hannah looks at me and shakes it—all the while the rest of the choir is singing the chorus. At the end of the song, Hannah shakes the bell into the little boy's ear, and he does the same with her. And *then, they hug! Hannah does not like to be touched due to her sensory processing disorder; however, she keeps her composure. The entire audience sighs, "Aww." I have never been more proud of my little girl. Christmas has come to town!*

A simple evening holiday program changed our routine and could have wreaked havoc. Children with autism require as much routine and structure as possible, and by definition, holidays and vacations are a break from routine activities. Holidays and vacations require adjustments to new places and generate a general anxiety about transitions and the unknown. Sometimes it goes unexpectedly smoothly, as it did the night of the choir event; other times, it's a disaster. As a result, it's critical to understand these stressors for our children, to prepare them and ourselves for celebrated holidays and more peaceful vacations. Be proactive so, later on, you won't need to be reactive in a difficult situation.

HOLIDAYS

Holidays spark nostalgic memories from my childhood that I would like to emulate for my own children. I vividly remember large gatherings at Grandma Diefenbach's for Christmas, formal Thanksgivings with all of the trimmings at Mom and Dad's, scouring the entire neighborhood on Halloween nights to fill my plastic pumpkin candy container before the jack-o-lanterns burned out, fireworks booming in our back yard to celebrate our nation's independence, my mother's tireless devotion to find every organized Easter egg hunt in the county, and countless birthday parties for my friends and me. Yes, I wanted to provide Hannah and Connor with the same extraordinary holiday celebrations that have always defined tradition for me; unfortunately, autism doesn't make that easy.

Holidays bring stress and anxiety to children with autism spectrum disorder. Routines and schedules are hard to maintain, and this lack of structure leaves Hannah disoriented and overwhelmed. New faces and places along with her sensitivities to touch and noise are too much to process—even at her current age. For these and other reasons, my daughter and I have suffered through some rough celebrations. Over the years, though, Hannah and I have implemented a number of coping strategies that allow her more enjoyment than ever before.

TIPS FOR THE HOLIDAYS

* ❖ If visiting family or friends, make sure there is a quiet, calm place for retreat.
* ❖ Practice unwrapping gifts ahead of time.
* ❖ Create a picture book for your child with the faces of the people your family is going to visit.
* ❖ Allow your child to eat preferred foods for holiday dinners and to be excused when finished.
* ❖ Consider writing a letter beforehand to your friends and family that you plan on visiting so they know what to expect.
* ❖ Gradually decorate your home for the holidays instead of completing all at once.

FORM A RETREAT ROOM

When she was only eighteen months, I determined that while visiting family in New York for the holidays, Hannah needed a room for retreat—a quiet space away from all of the commotion that would provide tools for sensory modulation; a calm in the storm. Before the celebration would begin, I'd place calming items in this retreat room: a bean bag chair, a Gertie ball (ball made of vinyl and used for anxiety due to its soft, tactile feel), Play-Doh, books, her iPad, a drawing pad with colored pencils, and Wikki Sticks (bendable, colorful strands used for creativity that are allergy-free).

Prior to establishing this retreat, Hannah would have meltdowns the moment the family started passing around and unwrapping Christmas gifts. The noise and happy chaos zapped all of her emotional resources.

She cried, even screamed multiple times with her hands placed over her ears. Now that I understand her sensory processing disorder, I alleviate holiday anxiety by creating a cushion of quiet, minimizing sound levels and any activity outside Hannah's control. We found it was even necessary to practice present-opening skills to lessen her anxiety.

TEACH HOW TO UNWRAP

Up until the age of five, people would hand Hannah a wrapped present, and she was at a loss for what to do. While people were opening their own presents, she simply wore a glazed look on her face. Her cousin, Peyton, only four months older, would patiently help Hannah. Hannah probably didn't understand the concept of gift receiving and opening. Plus, her fine motor challenges and the trouble she had with crossing midline made the motions required for pulling off wrapping paper and untying ribbons impossible. Looking back, I'm realizing she probably didn't even have the motor planning to know where to begin. Instead of trying, she just let the present sit beside her. She didn't watch others to copy what they did.

To help Hannah gain understanding and confidence, our occupational therapist bought inexpensive toys and wrapped them for Hannah. She gave them to Hannah and explained the concept, then walked her through each step needed to open a wrapped box or pull out the tissue from a gift bag. The Christmas following this "training," I snapped a photo of Hannah unwrapping a treasured gift—Saige, her American Girl doll. She's holding the large rectangular box high in the air in what I know is a pose of triumph. Others would infer she's happy with the doll. Maybe it's a lot of both!

INTRODUCE THE PEOPLE

When Hannah was two years old, our occupational therapist created a special picture book that contained snapshots of our relatives and closest friends. This book familiarized Hannah with individuals she might see at gatherings. Interestingly, that was not the book's original intent. We made the book when Hannah was nonverbal and we were trying to get Hannah to use her voice—we thought she might point and say people's names as we turned the pages of the book. It worked for that purpose; in fact, it led to her finally saying "Mommy." Repurposing the book as a holiday de-stressor and preparation tool worked well. She walked in seeing cousins and aunts who weren't once-a-year strangers but instead familiar faces she recognized right away.

LIMIT TIME AT THE TABLE

Even at twelve years old, Hannah cannot sit in a chair for an hour-long holiday dinner, trying new foods and listening to adults talk, and she certainly couldn't do that when she was a very young age. I didn't expect her to then, nor do I expect it of her now. No one would enjoy their meal if I did. I place her preferred foods on her plate and she knows she must try a little of each of the served foods. When Hannah has finished an acceptable amount of her dinner, she is excused. I admit, however, this has not always been the case.

At the beginning of a holiday meal with family, I used to pretend that everything was going to be okay. I would place small portions of the softer foods on Hannah's plate, and she would resist eating them. After she realized she wasn't going to be served her preferred foods with safe textures, she would cry and refuse to eat anything. Everyone around the table would then have a discussion, weighing in with their "expert" input on what would work. That's when I would retreat to the kitchen to get Hannah's preferred foods. By the time I returned, her hands would be covering her ears due to her hypersensitivity to sound, and she and I would then relocate to try to create a space where she could eat in peace.

Now, I realize I should have written both my family and my husband's family a letter when Hannah was around eighteen months old, explaining the challenges Hannah faced during holidays. They now understand, but earlier explanations might have helped the holidays run smoother and alleviate my self-inflicted guilt. As Hannah's mom, I felt her behavior in their presence was a reflection of my parenting. I would have included Hannah's dietary needs, sensory challenges, need for a retreat room, and behavior expectations that Hannah has a difficult time fulfilling. Whatever age your child is, write that letter. Help your family understand.

DECORATE IN STAGES

I decorate for the holidays little by little rather than all at once to avoid a sudden disruption in the look and feel of our home. I also encourage Hannah and Connor to help me decorate, and Hannah enjoys this, as it gives her some control over the timing and the choices of where things are placed and in what order. I have also learned that fewer decorations help her more easily accept changes to her environment.

SCHEDULE CHANGES

Holiday activities seem to pop up all the time and get added to our weekly schedule. Unexpected adjustments cause Hannah tremendous confusion, so I've learned to communicate each change as soon as possible. When she was little, I'd simply share the week's schedule and continue to repeat it to be sure she knew the order of activities. However, reinforcing a plan that doesn't go according to schedule can backfire. Autism has blessed Hannah with an amazing memory—miss a promised activity and expect repercussions.

As Hannah has grown older, I share my updated electronic calendar with her—she can look at it on her iPad, though this could easily be done with a physical calendar hanging in a communal space for her to study. I believe the up-to-date calendar adds a kind of structure to events outside her normal routine. This, too, helps lessen her holiday stress.

BIRTHDAYS

I have always gone big when celebrating my children's birthdays because my parents always did the same for my brother and me. However, birthdays aren't always easy for my daughter. I had planned to celebrate Hannah's fourth birthday at Chuck E. Cheese's. She had never been there, and I was still new enough to parenting a child with autism that I was certain she would enjoy all the rides, arcade machines, and the overhead maze.

I was lucky on that birthday to have only invited relatives. As soon as we walked into Chuck E. Cheese's Hannah covered her ears and screamed, "It hurts! It hurts!" Her eyes were twice as big as the arcade tokens, and her panic was increasing by the second. We turned around, rushed out the door, and drove home, celebrating in the quiet, familiar, calm environment of home where it didn't hurt.

OTHER PEOPLE'S RESPONSES

Most of the time, people have been kind and understanding of Hannah's needs. A few times, however, people who didn't know me felt free to judge me as a parent.

Thanksgiving 2007 was hectic. Hannah had been officially diagnosed with autism in February, and we were juggling multiple therapies and a plethora of doctor's appointments. Connor was born in March, and we cherished the thrill of watching him reach his developmental milestones—so different from his sister. I was teaching full-time and working on my gifted and talented licensure, and my husband had just undergone another administrative job change with a huge learning curve. We had a lot on our plates. In the midst of that, my in-laws called from New York to say they were coming to Indiana for Thanksgiving.

No way could we pull off a traditional meal at home. Instead, I made an executive decision to dine on a wonderful Thanksgiving feast catered at a local, upscale facility. This eliminated my preparation while keeping the event special at a time when Hannah was failing to thrive, upset that she had no means to communicate, and we were experiencing more frequent and intensifying meltdowns.

We arrived excited for our feast—a special treat we would normally never allow ourselves. To enjoy our meal, I had to focus Hannah's attention on something else: a Baby Einstein DVD. After being seated, I set up the portable DVD player and started the video. I then fed her the few spoonfuls of applesauce and yogurt she would eat and waited for our table to be called to the buffet. My back was to the buffet line when I heard, "Parents these days. And teachers wonder why our kids can't focus in school! Who can compete with that type of dynamic? How old do you think that little girl is? I just call it lazy parenting."

For a few moments I didn't turn around to see the woman's face. No one else in our family seemed to hear her. I held what the woman said to myself for a while, and then I just broke, feeling as fragile as the glass water goblet I'd been sipping from. I repeated the woman's words and our table fell silent for the rest of our meal. In that silence, I grew angry. After all, my husband and I were two educators. We always do what is best for kids—our own kids and all the kids we teach and lead every day at school.

How can she judge me? She doesn't even know me! Her audacity emboldened me to do something I shouldn't have done—especially on a holiday. But I had to.

I excused myself from our table, handed Connor to my husband, and walked over to the couple's table. "Excuse me," I said, "I am so sorry to interrupt your dinner, but I feel as if you interrupted mine. I owe you an explanation. When walking by our table you commented on my lazy parenting and how this type of parenting is affecting students in the classroom. I want you to know that I have been a classroom teacher for fourteen years and my husband is an assistant principal. Our daughter has a developmental delay called autism that makes it impossible for us to be out in public without a meltdown. Her therapies, our baby, and our jobs leave us so exhausted that we thought we would use the DVD player to calm her so we could enjoy a Thanksgiving meal. Not all situations are as they seem. Please be careful when judging others."

I turned and walked back to our table. Just as I arrived, the DVD finished and Hannah was crying because she noticed the noise level in the room, and Connor had just dropped another spoon from the table.

We left.

TRADITIONS OFFER HOLIDAY STRUCTURE

As I said, I prioritize building traditions into the kids' lives simply because I grew up with so many that I cherish. Traditions nourish our hearts and our souls, uniting a family to give roots. And while one of the biggest challenges of holidays is the way they throw off daily routines and patterns that our kids need, holiday traditions do offer something kids with autism cherish: structure.

Traditions make holidays special for everyone, offering something expected in the midst of all the unexpected disruption. At Christmas time, Hannah and Connor love to find Hermie Waldo (our Elf on the Shelf), decorate the tree, uncover their daily surprise trinkets hidden in the Advent calendar, hang their stockings, imagine themselves as a character in my Dickens village collection, listen to me read "A Visit from St. Nicholas," attend church service, and enjoy a drive through our neighborhood spying the glistening lights and illuminated yard displays.

On Thanksgiving, they want to write their blessings on homemade turkey feathers crafted from construction paper, watch the Macy's Thanksgiving Day Parade, hear the cranberries for the salad pop on the stove, and gather around the table with family (just not for long!).

On Halloween, they love to make jack-o-lanterns, choose their costumes, and trick-or-treat. Trick-or-treating is fun for Hannah even though the only candy she'll eat is Reese's peanut butter cups. Easter is about dressing up for the celebration at church, dyeing eggs, hunting for the eggs, and seeing what Grandma Ashley placed in their baskets.

I truly believe that holiday traditions provide cohesion to a family unit. Autism barely interferes with that. In fact, I think it's one of the best things for a child with autism, so bring on the traditions!

VACATIONS

My family traveled a lot when I was a child, so my childhood memories include the thrill of visiting faraway places. I want Hannah and Connor to have similar shared experiences and memories. We live in a country with exciting and beautiful destinations. Hannah and Connor need to see the national landmarks, jump in the ocean's waves, and experience the variety of museums.

When Hannah was eight years old and Connor was six, I started our family's fifty-state challenge. First, I bought the *National Geographic Kids Ultimate U.S. Road Trip Atlas*. The kids and I look through the atlas and choose the places we want to visit. In each state, we take family pictures at specific landmarks. On a large United States children's map that hangs in our office, we stick a pin in the landmark's location on the map, attach string to the pin, and attach the string with the date and location on the picture outside of the map. Sounds like a lot of fun, right? Well, it is. Most of the time. When autism is involved, a project like that can feel hijacked.

Vacations do seem to be a challenging, downright impossible feat for most families with children on the autism spectrum. Our experiences have revealed how I can better prepare for vacations by including essential components in my planning while eliminating adverse elements in the journey itself that cause anxiety to Hannah. Many incidents still occur that simply can't be prevented; however, we minimize incidents as much possible. I've learned to travel smarter because autism is involved, but I wasn't always so wise. In fact, I was blindsided early on with the challenge of vacations.

PLAYING BY HANNAH'S RULES

When Hannah was a baby, we took her on vacations all the time because the autism didn't present many problems—sure, she didn't want to be held or make eye contact, but she was a baby, so it didn't pose any issues on our trip. She didn't show any signs of heightened anxiety, no need for routine, nor any fear of the unknown. Then, when she turned four, we decided to take a weekend vacation with the four of us—a short weekend trip to Chicago, Illinois, about three and a half hours from home.

This was our first family vacation since Hannah's diagnosis two years prior, so we had no idea the impact it would have on her.

We were very excited to get to Chicago. My husband and I had planned to surprise the kids and stay at a hotel with themed rooms from Playhouse Disney (their favorite television network). Halfway to Chicago, Hannah grew anxious and angry. She was making muffled sighs and troubled moans, kicking the back of my seat, throwing toys, and flapping her hands. At the age of four, this was not typical car behavior for Hannah. We reminded her we were on vacation and listed all of the fun activities ahead: Shedd Aquarium, the Museum of Science and Industry, the LEGO Store, and the Rainforest Café.

Upon arrival at the hotel, the doorman showed Hannah the revolving doorway. Once in, she refused to step out. She screamed when I walked in to retrieve her. She kept running back to the revolving door. After a noisy check-in, we approached the elevator. Hannah then would not stop pressing the elevator buttons. She would get stuck on each repetitive behavior. When the elevator finally appeared, I swooped down to pick her up and put her into the elevator. She screamed, with a full elevator of people, all the way to floor sixteen, with frequent stops to allow people off. All I could do was cover her mouth with my hand. After exiting the elevator, I put Hannah down to help my husband with Connor and our luggage. While the rest of the family walked to our room, Hannah ran back to the elevator and continued her button-pushing ritual. After much coaxing, we were able to get Hannah, Connor, and all our luggage into our room. What was going on with Hannah?

After the kids enjoyed our themed room a while, we decided to take them a few blocks down and around the corner to the Disney Store. We would need to use the elevator again. The same thing happened getting on and off the elevator. Exiting the hotel, I opted to use the sliding glass doors this time instead of the revolving door. Hannah was used to these doors due to our visits to Riley Children's Hospital; however, it was clear she had no intention of following us. After chasing her for half a block, I decided to carry her. After a while, I let her down—a bad idea. Upset because she stepped on a line in the concrete sidewalk, she was determined to go back to the hotel and retrace her steps so she wouldn't step on any lines. To avoid a complete meltdown, my husband took her back. This time, they made it to the Disney Store without a problem. Once inside, she was unusually fascinated with walking the perimeter of the store as quickly as possible. I'm not even sure it registered to Hannah that we were in a children's wonderland.

We then walked to Gino's East Pizza, a legendary Chicago restaurant. It had been a while since lunch, and I knew that Hannah couldn't tolerate anything on the menu, so after the hostess seated us, I prepared the packed food Hannah would eat. Hannah continued to be agitated and refused to even touch her regular foods. We were disheartened beyond words. As we left, Hannah counted each of the twelve steps down the stairway—just as she had counted all twelve on the way to our table.

After returning to our hotel room, my husband and I were at an absolute loss for what to do. We stayed in the hotel that evening despite her continued anxiety and outbursts—and a concerned visit from the property's manager.

The next morning, we took a leap of faith that her behavior would improve. We hailed a taxi to take us to Shedd Aquarium. Hannah was not about to get in the taxi, so my husband got into the taxi with Connor, and I placed Hannah inside. She sprawled across both of our laps the entire way—screaming while we held her down. She needed normalcy—our vehicle, her car seat, and the routine seating arrangement. After a brief tour of Shedd Aquarium with Hannah—who refused to stay in her stroller but wandered off if she wasn't contained—we knew it was best for our vacation to be over. It was anything but a vacation. We headed home.

TIPS ON TRAVEL[14]

* Pre-plan by looking at pictures of your destination with your child.
* Create a visual schedule to help your child prepare for changes and transitions that may occur.
* Make sure to take items on the trip that will help your child feel more at home.
* Take a lot of reinforcing items: favorite foods, iPad, and favorite toys.
* Get a bracelet or a necklace for your child to wear that contains emergency information.
* Call ahead to your destination to see what accommodations they offer for people with special needs.

PLANNING AHEAD

It often feels like our family is governed by an arbitrary set of rules that no other family has to endure on their vacations. I know I'm not alone—children with autism struggle to cope while on vacations, so families all over the nation are having to retrace their steps to avoid stepping on lines and find ways to calm their child in a taxi or while touring a museum. I'm far enough along on our journey I can assure other parents they can do several things to make trips easier. With each vacation, I get smarter and Hannah's anxiety lessens. I've learned specific, worthwhile preparations I can make long before leaving for a vacation. Steal my ideas.

The first and most helpful process to prepare Hannah for a vacation is to show her brochures or websites of our destination. The more she knows about the place we're headed, the more comfortable she feels in the new environment. Maps of the property's layout are extremely helpful, so she can figure out how to navigate the space before she's in it. She also feels vested in the destination if she has had some say in the chosen activities. A prepared but loose schedule adds structure to her day, and structure helps every kid with autism. Hannah has helped plan schedules and activities for destinations like St. Louis, Disney World, Myrtle Beach, Gulf Shores, Milwaukee, and King's Island (an amusement park near Cincinnati, Ohio).

I frequently call ahead and see if our destinations offer anything to help our visit run more smoothly, because some destinations have special accommodations for children with special needs. I once asked Hannah's pediatrician to write a letter to the airline we were using that stated her diagnosis and specific challenges. This cut down on wait time getting on and off our flights. As Hannah has gotten older, I have found that handing the airline personnel a letter works better than talking about my daughter's challenges in front of her.

I always pack items that will help Hannah feel more at home: a pillow, her journal, a favorite stuffed animal and books, her sleep mask, and a picture of her beloved cat, Marshmallow. Along with comfort items, I also bring favorite foods, an iPad with her favorite movies and apps, and inexpensive new items purchased at a party store or dollar store, like miniature Rubik's Cubes and activity pads, to reinforce good behavior.

When Hannah was younger, I made sure that on vacations she wore a laminated card safety-pinned to her shirt that contained her name, diagnosis, our names, and our phone numbers. We also used the GPS bracelet and the Mommy I'm Here child locator, in case she took off running.

When Hannah was five years old, we took the kids to Great Wolf Lodge, a hotel and indoor water park. Thankfully, Hannah has always been an amazing swimmer because of aquatic therapy. While we walked into the water park and looked for a place to store our things, Hannah took off. It took the both of us ten minutes to find Hannah in the vast area. She had no care in the world about where we were, about getting lost, or even about getting into trouble. Even today, at the age of twelve, I struggle to get Hannah to stay with us— but these days she's too old for the Mommy I'm Here locator, and she's no longer at risk for running. These days she simply gets lost in her thoughts and then realizes she's not with us. Instead of panicking and learning the lesson of staying with us, she blames me for "losing" her. One day, I hope she'll learn the importance of staying close by.

KEEP IT SIMPLE

We learned not to pack too many excursions into one vacation. Moving from location to location leaves no time for the slow, smooth transitions that Hannah craves. **Cognitive flexibility** definitely isn't one of her strengths. She moves at her own pace. Planning fewer activities and taking breaks at the hotel allow for more structure and sensory breaks—we end up enjoying each other more at this slower pace (I actually think this is ideal for all children, not just those with autism).

JUST US

Although I really enjoy traveling with other families, it upsets Hannah's routine and structure even more than the outing would with just us. She's not used to handling the 24/7 presence of another family and the accompanying noise level, although she's usually the one making the noise. She needs time to be alone and quiet. Even simply sharing a vehicle with another family—including the people, conversations, luggage, snacks, and games—results in more frequent meltdowns. It's too much input for someone who struggles with a sensory processing disorder, and the last thing Hannah wants to do is to have a meltdown with people outside her immediate family. Plus, I want to avoid continually needing to apologize for her behavior. It feels as if I am continually being judged by my reactions to Hannah's meltdowns, even though I'm sure this isn't the case. We tried this multiple-family vacation setup once. I resolved never to put any of us, including the other family, in that situation again.

We have found another alternative that does work. It costs more and some of the convenience is lost, but we once caravanned with another family to Disney World and stayed in different hotel rooms. This worked because Hannah had more room traveling with less noise and was able to retreat to a quiet place in our hotel room in the evenings. However, as a single mom, one of the advantages of traveling in the same vehicle and staying in the same room with another family was cost efficiency and a road trip for moms and kids only. So that was a rare luxury.

COUNTDOWN

Hannah appreciates a monthly calendar to count down the days until vacation. She's challenged with the concept of time. Time is continuous with no boundaries, and it's not something that an individual can feel. A couple of years ago we used a free wall calendar, and every morning she woke up and checked off the day with a big red marker. Last year the kids and I even made a paper chain for the countdown and draped it across the mantle, tearing off one link of the chain every morning. Every time we ripped off a link, I discussed a few more details about the trip to make Hannah feel more comfortable, though the information helped Connor build anticipation, as well.

ANTICIPATE PROBLEMS

Before leaving for each of our trips, I try to brainstorm possible challenges we may face. Between the ages of four and eight, loud noises created sensory turmoil for Hannah, so I thought through each location and imagined the noise level and what I could do to minimize it. By choosing to enter a children's museum later in the day, fewer kids were around shrieking and laughing. Now that Hannah is twelve years old, loud noises no longer bother her except when added to other sensory obstacles. To address that, I always bring earplugs to places like amusement parks.

Hannah often wants to do things first, so I set the expectation that she and Connor will alternate turns the entire vacation—if either child brings it up, he or she will go last. This works well for both kids, because the discussion took place before we ever left home.

PACK FOOD

As I have mentioned, like most people on the spectrum, Hannah does not care for many foods, so I bring as many of her favorites as possible. Hannah has a weak sense of hunger. This magnifies her challenging behavior without her even realizing the cause—when her body needs fuel, she feels nervous and acts bossy, but doesn't recognize why. I always pack small containers of applesauce, bananas, cereal bars, fruit snacks, and peanut butter and jelly sandwiches for her. These are all convenient to place into a small backpack without a mess.

STAYING BACK

Some families may struggle with this idea, but I find it's easier on Hannah and on me sometimes to travel without her. Vacations are often so draining for kids with autism; it can be better not to put them through the transitions, environmental changes, and anxiety of the unknown. Though it's bittersweet, they may be happier staying back, and as parents, we can enjoy a trip without the added strain of anticipating our child's needs. When you have a situation where you trust they are staying with a loved one who is aware of their needs and will engage them in their preferred activities, you can travel without guilt. In fact, their siblings may also need, deserve, and appreciate this special time having their parents all to themselves.

For all the things about autism that chafe our family vacations, we do choose to travel together most often. It makes me feel more normal, as I refuse to allow autism to limit our family more than it already has. I rejoice in seeing Hannah jump in the ocean waves, when everything about our family feels normal for a day. Seeing Hannah uninhibited and laughing without anxiety feels like a miracle. My heart calms. I've lounged at a pool in Myrtle Beach and heard my daughter on the deck with the DJ belting out the latest Taylor Swift song—these moments shock me into happiness. I permanently want to hold these scenes in my mind.

They make up for the other times—like the intense discomfort she feels when someone accidentally gets too close to her in line for an amusement ride and she lets them know, or when she has no discernment to stay with me at the Most Magical Place on Earth (which steals the "magic" from the Magic Kingdom). We muddle through each uncomfortable predicament and try to find a solution or let it go.

Your expectations change for vacations, as they do for everything, and what used to bother you simply doesn't anymore. It does take a while to get to that point. But you do. You will.

It's not about us as parents, and our kids aren't bad. We face the challenge of dealing with a mismatch between the environment and our kids' coping abilities. I can only control so much about vacations and autism, so I will face issues; however, I don't let my dread of issues keep us from heading off on adventures. It's worth all the planning and phoning to expose my children to the great locations and opportunities our country has for kids to play and learn and grow.

Two years ago, while once again vacationing in Chicago, we were walking down the Magnificent Mile. Hannah and Connor saw a huge splash pad for kids at Millennium Park. They asked if they could run and dance in the water. My first thought was, *Of course not. There are still about five blocks before even reaching our hotel. We don't have a jacket or dry clothes with us, and we would need to get ready all over again before going out to dinner.*

Then I thought, *What would be more breathtaking than both of my kids dancing, playing, jumping, and running through the water show right now?*

I said yes.

The look on both of their faces when they ran through the water spoke of freedom from worries as they stepped outside of their boxes.

Inspirational writer Vivian Greene says, "Life is not just about waiting for the storm to pass—you have to learn to dance in the rain." My prayer for my daughter is that there will be a lot more dancing in her future.

ᙣᘓᕟᙣᘓ **Wisdom from the Round Table** ᙣᘓᕟᙣᘓ

Lori R.: I will never forget the first time I let Cameron drive a go-cart by himself in Pigeon Forge, Tennessee. That, in itself, made the vacation. It was a victory to be celebrated!

Jen: Prepare your child as much as you can for what is coming next. Schedules are very helpful. Noah also has a calendar that hangs on our garage door. Anything scheduled that is not routine for Noah goes on that calendar—vacations included. I also pack Noah's favorite snacks, DVD player with DVD's, iPad, and fidget toys.

Lori V.: I've always tried to do things early in the morning or when I think crowds are at their lowest. Overstimulation and long lines cause Byron problems.

Susan: There is no vacation when you have a child with autism. You are either changing your schedule to accommodate your child, or if you leave them with someone you are constantly worried about them.

Karen: We had to take several precautions to make sure our boys were safe while on vacations because it was as if they didn't know danger.

Sarah: A specific agenda before the vacation allows Mitchell time to understand the upcoming transitions. We also remind him that the plans may need to change. If he feels he would rather stay back, we allow him to do so.

CHAPTER NINE

flying solo

Single Motherhood

How partners approach the particular stresses of raising an autistic child may determine whether their relationship is stretched to the breaking point—or, ultimately, solidified.

—Sigan Hartley

June 2013

I closed on our new home alone on Friday. I was scared to sign on a mortgage for that amount only on my teacher's salary. Friends and family members helped me move in the evening. Hannah and Connor played on the driveway while they waited for their dad to pick them up for the weekend. One of my friends had her high school son, Chris, come to help, and Chris brought one of his friends. The boy didn't know my family whatsoever. I believe that's why his comment, while he hauled boxes to the U-Haul, shocked me so. He said, "Does anyone else hear that little girl in the driveway talking? You know who she sounds like? She sounds like Sheldon Cooper's girlfriend on The Big Bang Theory*!" I guess you don't have to be a doctor to uncover her autism.*

As the garage door on our new home slowly rises, it unveils a gorgeous Sunday. I cross the street with only my old house keys in hand.

As I walk five houses down, I believe I'm ready to say goodbye to the house that had become our home after Hannah's diagnosis in 2006. As a newborn, Connor was brought here over six years ago. It really is time to move on—no other option. The three of us don't need such a large home, and I wouldn't be able to afford the mortgage. So proud of my new beginning, but nostalgic for a past that could have been. I've stretched the truth by telling the kids how much better our new home will be. I had to make a sad situation better for them.

My husband and I separated in September of 2011, and our divorce was final earlier this year. Every soul fiber in me screamed with pain. Not something I ever wanted to happen—no one ever wins in divorce. I've been told that kids are resilient in matters like these—it will make them stronger, they say.

Will it? And why do they have to be stronger? I've heard all the positive spins on bad things that happen to good kids, but I still don't buy them. Yes, I understand how these experiences build maturity, resilience, and flexibility. At what price? Wouldn't they be made stronger emotionally going to bed with both of their parents under the same roof? Wouldn't they build maturity through continuity, instead of having to face the "switching hour," a term I've had to learn: It's the time and experience of leaving one parent's home in order to be in the other parent's home at intervals decided by the parents or the court. How is that going to work out well for them? How is it positive to worry if the materials needed for a school assignment are available at the parent's house where you're going to be doing your homework for the next day? Divorce creates those scenarios for any child—now one of my children has to add autism's need for structure and routine on top of that!

How I hope and pray "they" are right, those experts who promise they'll bounce back and grow strong instead of descending into anxiety and fear.

I longed to keep our family together, but marriage takes two. I felt waylaid by the demise of our marriage. Sometimes all you have left is gratitude for what you really do have—and that is two amazing kids and a mother who would do anything for them. My hope is that they always know how much I love them and they walk through the rest of their life knowing I'll always be there for them any way I can. My kids will make it because I am making it!

I unlock the front door and walk in. I look up the staircase and am reminded that Hannah will no longer be counting those same seventeen steps as she paces up and down. I walk up the steps, counting each one, and head straight to her room. Her initials, HGT, still remain on the wall. I'll never forget reading her favorite books, You Are My I Love You *and* Goodnight Moon, *in this very room.* Goodnight stars. Goodnight air. Goodnight voices everywhere.

As I walk into Connor's room, I picture him as a young toddler, standing up in his crib while bending and straightening his legs, yearning to be released—and that magical grin blowing raspberries until he was set free. I can't stand the nostalgia and journey back downstairs.

Most of Hannah's therapy occurred here in the family room. I recall the speech therapist with the duck hand puppet that would quack to entice Hannah to open her mouth to speak. And the occupational therapist with the magnetic pole that attached to the puzzle pieces which encouraged Hannah to cross midline; the developmental therapist who urged Hannah to string the beads, hammer the pegs, and blow the bubbles.

The office offers more memories: Hannah's time on starfall.com—basically teaching herself to read. The toy box she hid behind in order to dodge dinner, and the holes in the wall that once housed the screws to Hannah's bulletin board that read "Hannah's School News"—my organizational system for keeping track of all three preschools in one place.

I leave the office and walk past the dining room table—how many times I either forced Hannah back into her seat or begged her to just take a small bite, to pick up the spoon or simply grab the food itself, and place it into her mouth without any texture sensitivity or gag reflex. Just one bite. How many months did she push that miniature shopping cart around the kitchen island backward before she finally let go? That infamous LeapFrog Fridge Phonics magnetic letters set stuck to the fridge. Time and time again she would line those letters up and then place them one by one into the device that would sing, "The A says ah, and A says ae. Every letter makes a sound. The A says ah and ae."

Looking out at the play set, I'll miss the time spent playing with the kids in our backyard. This past year, Connor and I enjoyed our own special time in the playhouse above the green slide. He would pretend to be a pirate steering the ship with the large yellow wheel while I stood on the slide and pleaded his mercy as his dupe on the plank. I laugh when I realize what the neighbors probably thought.

I decide it's time to leave the keys for the new owner, and I exit through the laundry room. I didn't have the time to appreciate how nice our home really was. I had more important things to be concerned with. Yes, this is sad. But I can't allow myself to give these emotions any weight right now. I have my memories, and we're blessed with a new beginning up the street!

Yes, my marriage did become part of that noxious statistic published time and time again—80 percent of marriages that have a child with autism do not survive.[15] My husband left when Hannah was in first grade and Connor was in preschool. However, I don't believe divorce is inevitable. Does autism add pressures to a marriage? Sure, it adds emotional, financial, and time strains, but marriages are not doomed when an autism diagnosis is introduced to the family. As for that infamous, even terrifying statistic, some experts argue the validity of that 80 percent.[16] I've researched the topic, identified my own marriage's pitfalls, and spoken with other couples who raised children with autism while enjoying lasting relationships. My conclusion? Don't allow your child's autism to be your scapegoat! Divorce is not inevitable, nor can autism be blamed for the collapse of a marriage.

Dr. Barry Prizant echoes the same conclusion in his book, *Uniquely Human*. He writes, "What we do know is that stresses in a relationship cause divorce. Raising a child with a disability can be stressful. If there are already cracks in the foundation of a marriage, then having a child with autism adds additional pressure, and that could lead to divorce. But it's never the lone factor."

In my daughter's second official autism diagnosis evaluation, the doctor wrote: "An obvious strength for this little girl is her intact family, who seem to be very dedicated to her future development and success." After the divorce, this statement riddled me with guilt. While I was still dedicated to her future development and success, our family was no longer intact. When I found myself a single mother and primary caregiver to two children—not to mention Hannah's unofficial caseworker—I didn't feel strong. I felt I was barely keeping my head above water, but I grew and found ways to stay dedicated to Hannah's future development and success, just as the doctor wrote. And somehow I managed to carve out a life for myself as well.

So if you do find yourself in my place, and I pray you don't, I hope my strategies and work ethic encourage you to aim for balance and efficiency in your life. If you're still married, and I hope you are, you may still get ideas to create a healthier life for yourself. After all, many of my happily married friends tell me the majority of the labor generally falls on one parent anyway—so, married or not married, you're carrying a heavy burden similar to that of a single mom. We can do this. We need hope . . . and ideas.

MARRIAGE

I don't watch much television, but I happened to catch and record *The Oprah Winfrey Show* on autism in April 2007. That episode touched and taught me more about the topic than anything I'd been privy to beforehand. One mother's interview in particular hit close to home. Michele Pierce Burns said, "Having a child who needs what my son, Danson, needs made it very difficult for me to balance my life—to be a mother, have a job, and be a wife. I didn't give that marriage what I could've because I had nothing left to give."[17]

I had nothing left to give.

I wanted to apply her wisdom to our situation. I wanted to do everything I could for Hannah, but still have enough to give to my marriage.

REACTIONS TO THE DIAGNOSIS

You may recall from chapter 1 that my husband and I had different reactions to the autism diagnosis. I felt a lot of guilt. I seriously thought

I had done something to cause Hannah's autism. I often mourned in the middle of the night, waking my husband. Then, I went into caseworker mode trying to make a difference in my daughter's life. I wanted to prove the neurologist's prognosis wrong. And during all of those demands, I birthed an amazing little boy, continued my own education, and taught full-time.

My husband was and still is a good father, but he was embarrassed by the diagnosis at first. His way of grieving looked different than mine. While Hannah's autism was something that I couldn't stop talking about, it was something he didn't want to discuss outside of listening to my worries. This happens often. Liane Kupferberg Carter discusses a similar experience between her and her husband in her book *Ketchup is My Favorite Vegetable: A Family Grows Up With Autism*. Carter quotes her husband's words: "I don't want you talking about it to all your friends. Don't tell anyone. I don't want anyone to look at him differently." If looking for a memoir spanning decades with a family's experience with autism, I highly recommend Liane Kupferberg Carter's book.

Our dramatically different griefs created bitterness and resentment in our marriage. It was difficult to turn to one another for support. I wanted to hear that everything was going to be okay, but he couldn't promise me that. He wanted me to appreciate his need for withdrawal, but I saw it as him sticking his head in the sand and, quite frankly, weak. Once again, hindsight is 20/20 and I probably shouldn't have been so quick to judge; however, I had no time for withdrawal. The clock was ticking down. In other words, each of us felt the other should be doing something differently.

SHARING RESPONSIBILITIES

My husband's demanding and stressful job as an assistant principal required long hours. To make matters worse, each of the schools where he worked during our marriage were at least forty minutes from our new home. This wasn't his fault—assistant principal jobs are hard to get. However, solo parenting wore on me. I faced the monotony and tension of therapy mostly alone, watching Hannah challenged all evening with skills that made her feel uncomfortable and bracing myself for the therapists' questions about what we'd worked on since the last session. I layered onto myself guilt upon guilt. And then, when the last therapy session wrapped up, I'd fix dinner alone and hope that just once Hannah wouldn't vomit the tiny bit of food I managed to coax into her mouth.

I felt so alone, but I now know I wasn't the only mom dealing with these pressures on my own. So many parents of children with autism are doing it all in hopes of saving their children. What parent wouldn't? But we're prone to stress, anxiety, depression, and self-doubt. Studies show that we have as much cortisol in our brains as active-duty military members and we could develop post-traumatic stress disorder equal to that of a combat soldier.[18] However, the couples I interviewed whose marriages survived and flourished after a diagnosis all had one thing in common—they changed their family's dynamics. A change in dynamics helped them adjust to the barrage of therapy and doctor appointments.

Parents hear about monumental improvements in individual cases and begin the treadmill of therapies in hopes that their child will have similar results. If he doesn't, they feel as if they haven't tried hard enough and that there must be another therapy that will be their magic bullet. We must explore options to get our children opportunities for growth to emerge as far as they can, while also possibly changing the dynamics of our household to allow for our children's stringent schedule. We must also avoid the temptation to push and push when we see we've reached maximum potential; however, remember that accomplishments can take time.

It's hard to find a balance of doing all we can without knocking ourselves out, and it's not clear why some children with autism seem to get over the most egregious aspects of autism and some don't. So we do our best, and those of us who must do it all on our own, flying solo, will rely on others for help if our spouse is unable or unwilling to step up.

As discussed in chapter 4, Hannah had a rigorous therapy schedule and an ambitious team of therapists. My schedule conformed to Hannah's schedule, and if she wasn't in therapy, I was checking therapy bills, scheduling therapy, corresponding with providers, or trying to get her to eat. I felt as if I was on a singular journey with her and her autism while tending to Connor's needs and making sure I didn't miss out on precious time with him. Notice how I say I felt? I was not really on a singular journey, as Hannah's father appreciated my work with Hannah. He attended therapies and doctors' appointments when his schedule permitted. But it felt as though he got up early and went to work, abandoning me to the care for our two children, leaving me to manage the multitude of appointments. I got up thirty minutes later, dressed and fed Hannah and Connor, packed their needed materials, sang shape and number songs in the car for Hannah's benefit, dropped them at daycare, taught a full day, picked the kids up from daycare, and then participated in one or two therapies by the time he made it home for dinner.

I also did the laundry and solved domestic emergencies like the time the Bradford pear tree fell on the play set, or the day the backup sump pump failed to kick in, or when the hot water heater leaked in our basement to give me a heads-up it needed to be replaced. I was the only one home, so I dealt with everything mostly by myself. My husband would return my calls, emails, and texts when he was available. He would also try to help meet with the occasional serviceman. Over time, I learned that I just needed to do it myself. No wonder I was running on empty. My immune system was so low I'd catch every cold, flu, or pink eye going around our school. Iron levels proved to be fine, despite thinning hair. And at one appointment, my dentist accused me of chewing rocks in my sleep. I felt as if I was solely responsible for holding our household together. I couldn't find another way. My family needed my physical and mental health, but it seemed as if I was the only one pulling everyone else along.

I felt contempt and resentment. What a comfort to hear this sentiment echoed in a *Parenthood* episode where the character Kristina, the mom who has a child with autism, attends a parents' autism support group. One of the members shared that she felt deep resentment. Though the character was fictional, hearing someone else confess her dark struggle validated my emotions.[19] You can find information on the episode in the endnotes; I highly recommend watching it.

In the early days I didn't realize the scope of the saying *autism is a diagnosis for the entire family* because I was so consumed with responsibilities that I didn't realize how it was straining our marriage. However, my own broken marriage serves as a warning that if we don't allow the diagnosis to change our lifestyle for the better, the diagnosis may adversely affect other areas of life. Looking back, our family would have benefited from my taking a year or two off work and my husband waiting to take an administrative position. My friend Lori suggested this for me, and I should've given it more consideration and weight. Family trumps everything else. We believed that in our heads, but in practice we thought we could do it all. And we did. But by the time we realized we couldn't love our family and live at the pace our work required, it was too late. The do-it-all mindset cost us our marriage.

Draw boundaries!

At the risk of sounding hypocritical, we special needs parents really need to pace ourselves and work with our spouses to share in the responsibilities. This strengthens the bond of mutual appreciation. Communicate your needs and listen to your spouse without scorn or contempt. I continue to fiercely advocate the need for intense early intervention to maximize progress (a bigger payoff), but I also realize Hannah's therapy regimen was extremely aggressive. You must have time as a family to breathe. I also have found that the window of opportunity for growth never really closes. It just takes longer for our children to pick up the skills, and if we for whatever reason need to slow the pace, our children will still find ways to emerge. Hannah had time that I didn't believe existed, and so does your child. I know it doesn't seem like it, but they do! Take care of yourself, so you can take care of your family.

LOOKING BACK AT CONNECTING

My husband and I did spend alone time together when we were married. We tried to do something special every once in a while—we even took two vacations to Florida with just the two of us. But we should have taken more—and longer—trips together. Our vacations weren't frequent enough to truly connect as a couple, and they weren't long enough to recharge from total exhaustion. Learn from our mistake and take trips.

Also schedule dates as you would any other appointment or outing—they are the most important! The dates don't have to include anything too costly and the vacations don't have to be luxury destinations. Going for a cup of coffee or glass of wine, or even taking a walk is good for a date, and if you know how to find a deal on local lodging, you could enjoy a staycation to spend focused time together without spending a lot of money. Just make sure it's a chance to reconnect. This was not the focus of our dates. Instead, we erroneously spent our only alone time together discussing the kids, our schedules, career demands, and financial matters. At the time it seemed like the important stuff— and in a way, it was. But our marriage might have improved if we'd limited the time we spent talking through those topics and devoted plenty of time to laugh and enjoy each other.

ASK FOR HELP

Exemplary caregivers are essential for our children while married couples work. We had two top-notch, in-home daycare providers—I always said that they helped us raise our children. However, because we both worked outside of the home, we didn't ask for much help at any other time beyond date nights. We basically leaned on one another—there wasn't much time to organize anything else. That would have taken additional effort and we were depleted.

Again, my closest friend and teaching partner, Lori, has always been an emotional rock for our family, but we never actually asked her or anyone to help with groceries, cooking, laundry, or mowing. We should have. These days I'd be able to turn to online grocery services, cooking preparation workshops, and Amazon—in fact, I encourage married couples and single parents to take advantage of every new service that can simplify life. If your family can afford it, consider hiring a young kid in your neighborhood to weed and mow your lawn. Extended family members may also be able and willing to help out. My husband's family lived in New York and mine lived four hours away, so this wasn't an option for us, but if you've got family nearby who are able and willing, ask.

We did have someone clean our home once a month. I always kept our home picked up and organized, but to have someone do the deep cleaning was worth the money. I'd also prepare meals she could place in the crock pot to be ready for us that night. During the summer, we hired two sisters a few days a week to join the kids and me on outings to parks, museums, and the pool. Two extra sets of hands along with their boundless energy eased my load and increased fun for my kids—a few years later, when those sisters applied for jobs, colleges, and scholarships, they appreciated my letters of recommendation.

ADAPTABILITY AND FLEXIBILITY

If you and your spouse are able to change lifestyles and routines that have been intact for sometimes decades, you'll end up with a stronger marriage in the end. Try to accept that life is not the same, but it's going to be okay—your family unit is still together. Become resourceful and tolerate differences in emotions to avoid hurting each other's feelings. No one wants to feel alone with autism—take a thirty-minute timeout with one another on the porch. You say you don't have time? Take the time. Be flexible enough to support one another. A few of the Women from the Round Table have cited that embracing a strong spiritual life has also helped them, so if you enjoy a shared faith, find unity in your beliefs.

GET COUNSELING

Couples must get counseling at first signs of distress. We didn't do this until our marriage had already crumbled. By the time I was able to get my husband to join me in counseling he had already checked out of our marriage—he had mentally moved on before I had time to process the loss. My efforts to help proved futile. I reached out to his friends and a religious leader, but I believe those gestures only further upset him, as I wasn't allowing him time to withdraw. People handle anxiety in different ways. In time, I learned that individuals can't always control how grief manifests itself. So, in some families this could be a role reversal where the wife drops into a funk and the husband is lost and unable to get through to get her the help she needs because she refuses it. What do you do as the sole witness to a loved one's misery?

While it's too late for me, I did seek advice for you from our family's counselor, Dr. Jason Warner. Dr. Warner said that the dynamics between a husband and wife's relationship often take a back seat after their child receives an autism diagnosis. This poses emotional challenges between the couple. Though difficult to balance, Dr. Warner recommends spouses find common ground in sharing responsibilities or temporarily change the dynamics of the family during early interventions. According to Dr. Warner, couples who are not on the same page or who disagree with the course of interventions will suffer enormous strains within their relationship. He believes that the primary caregiving parent's life is indefinitely placed on hold, and the individual may lose him or herself, while the spouse with fewer caregiving responsibilities continues to live life as usual, but feels less integral to the marriage and family as they once were.

Sometimes a stranger who has worked with families that have a loved one on the spectrum can calm the perfect storm that surrounds emotions, finances, treatment decisions, division of labor, depression, lifestyle changes, and more. Finding a good mental health professional is as good as gold.

MARRIAGE TIPS FOR PARENTS
RAISING A CHILD WITH AUTISM[20]

❖ Remember that everyone reacts differently to an autism diagnosis.
❖ Take time to adjust to work/lifestyle changes that occur.
❖ Find time to be together as a couple.
❖ Ask for help from friends, family, or caregivers.
❖ Don't let one partner carry too much of the daily responsibilities.
❖ Get counseling.

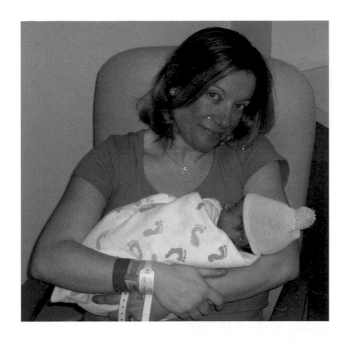

On Hannah's birth day, I was blessed to hold her close—as this wouldn't last long.

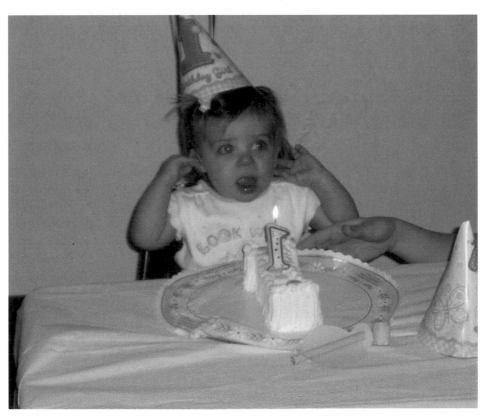

Hannah wouldn't tolerate the party hat's string touching her skin.

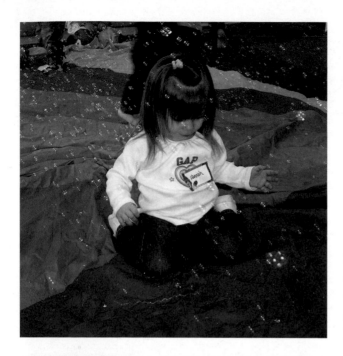

Hannah was in her own world and wouldn't interact with others at Gymboree Play and Music.

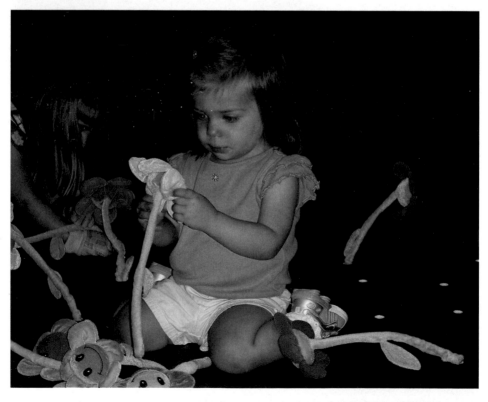

Hannah had no idea that she was supposed to be placing the flowers' stems into the holes. She continued to use the W-sitting position.

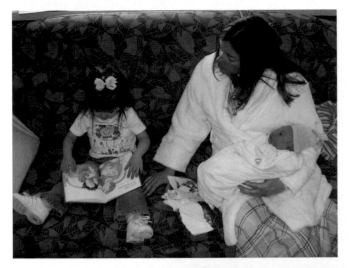

The day after Connor's birth, Hannah had been in the room for thirty minutes and hadn't looked at her brother once. This scene follows my crying episode with the chaplain.

Laquita (ST) had a dynamic personality while pulling Hannah's motor planning along in order to allow her to one day speak.

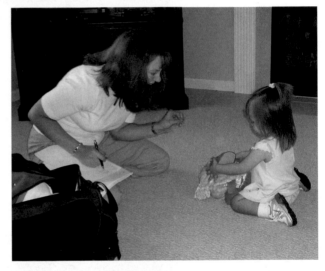

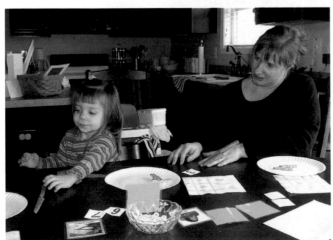

Tara (OT) used a variety of methods to encourage Hannah's feeding.

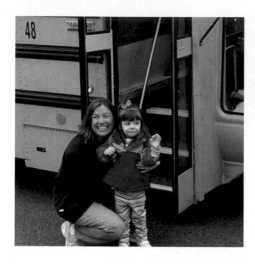

Hannah's first day of developmental preschool proved more stressful for me.

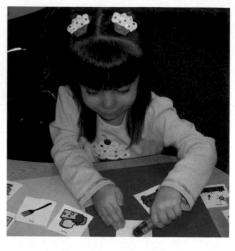

Hannah held it together at school, while home was a different story.

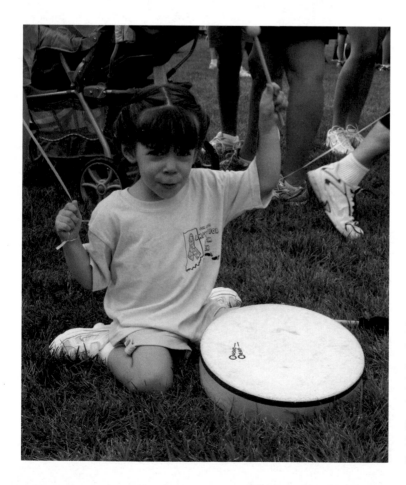

Hannah and the drum that entertained her while our team was gathering for heartfelt support.

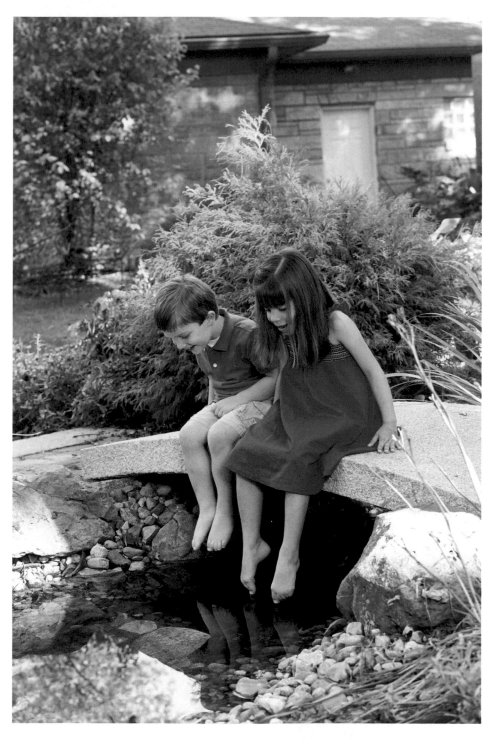

A rare expression of normalcy which I wish would've been the
norm, but wasn't.
Hanke Photography Inc.—Michelle Hanke

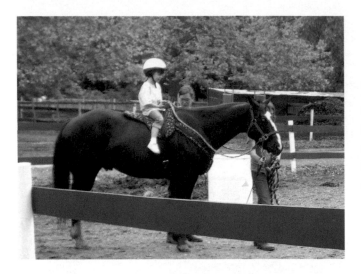

Molly and Magic (equine-assisted therapy) played an integral role in Hannah's emergence.

Whether in front of a crowd or on her piano in our home, music is a great escape for Hannah.

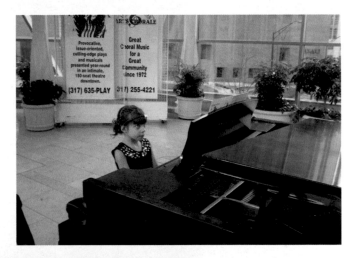

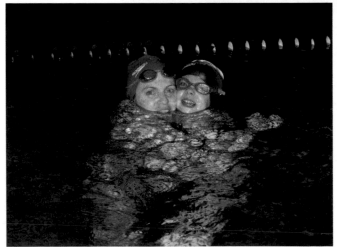

Katinka (aquatic therapy) realized the difference water could make for Hannah's sensory awareness. She hugged, smiled, and looked me in the eyes!

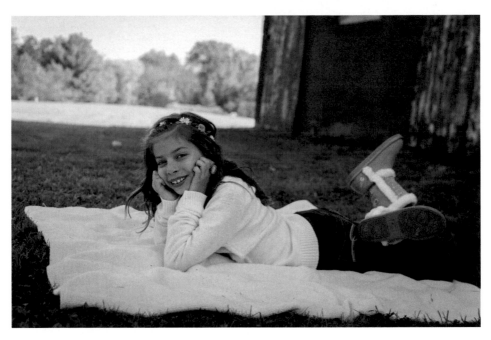

Hannah finds peace and comfort in nature like no other.
Ardea Photo—Andrea Moberly

My favorite vacation spot
with Hannah and Connor is Disney's Polynesian Village Resort.

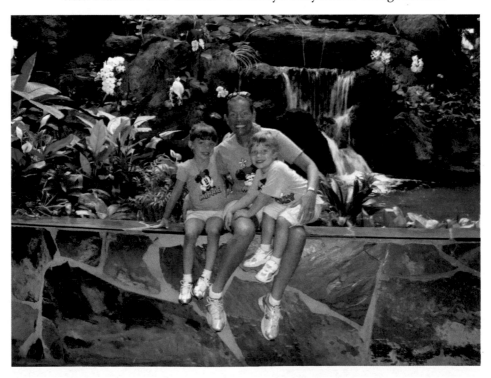

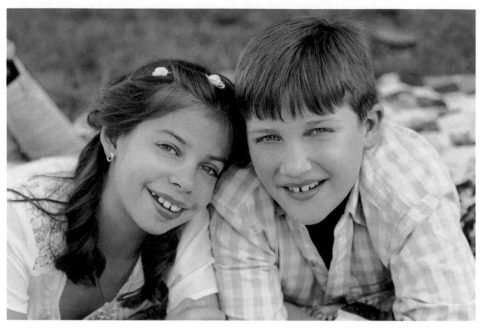

While they are two different individuals, their past, present, and future will
be inherently entwined as siblings.
Loree Alayne Photography—Loree Alayne Wheeler

Hannah's unconditional support and acceptance—friendships!
Ardea Photo—Andrea Moberly

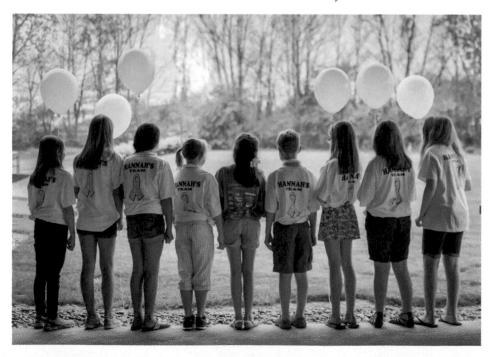

DIVORCE

I'll never forget having to tell Hannah and Connor that their dad and I would no longer be living in the same home. As my pastor counseled me, I told them that we loved both of them very much and this was in no way their fault.

"You have a very good mommy and daddy," I said, "but together we don't make one another better people." I told them none of us needed to be unhappy anymore, but I knew I would be unhappy for a long, long time.

Devastated, I lost the love of my life, stood in court to gain custody of the kids, and moved—all while maintaining an intensive therapy schedule for Hannah and holding down my full-time teaching position. I survived, and my children are thriving. I believe God closes some doors because it's time to move on. I wouldn't have moved on unless the circumstances forced me. I was not what my husband needed to live a joy-filled life; hence, he couldn't provide that for us, either. I do believe since our divorce he spends more quality time with our children. And it gets to be on his terms. At one time we did live a joy-filled life, however, and out of that joy-filled period came two remarkable children that neither divorce nor autism can taint or diminish. They remind me of the goodness we once enjoyed. I thought the divorce was going to break me—in the end, it woke me.

Harboring hurtful feelings only hurts those harboring them, and I deserve peace. But I face inevitable losses. I wish we would have remained a happy family—I'd rather wear a wedding ring and belong with someone. I dislike knowing that when I do start dating again, my children will probably feel awkward and confused. It also pains me when I hear people say that divorce is not an option for them. They don't realize it wasn't an option for me either—I was determined to make our marriage work but couldn't stop the divorce from happening. And being single doesn't make me or anyone else less of a person. If you're married and interacting with a single mom, remember that. And remember that if you're single and feeling like a second-class citizen. It's disappointing when reality contradicts your ideal.

I used to be thrown off by the idea that Hannah and Connor would not spend every night in our home and felt troubled knowing they were having experiences I knew nothing about and couldn't share. I soon learned to be happy my children were having new experiences—whether I was with them or not. It's hard enough that their parents are divorced—they don't need the Spanish Inquisition when returning home.

Hannah and Connor spend every other weekend with their father and Wednesday evenings overnight with him. Hannah painfully describes their situation, "Connor and I feel like peanut butter and jelly smashed between two pieces of bread." That was difficult to hear. Due to Hannah's autism, the court wanted to be sure this arrangement would work. I feared it would upset Hannah's routine and wreak havoc on us all, so the judge appointed a guardian ad litem (GAL) to monitor the outcome of her ruling for a short period of time. The GAL interviewed my husband and me individually along with our daycare provider, Hannah's teacher, and the school's guidance counselor. I felt so degraded and humbled during this interview. After all I had done for my daughter, I felt like I was being grilled by Child Protective Services (CPS). The GAL was courteous and respectful, but the interactions left me shaken, wondering why I had to be evaluated to determine the amount of time I could spend with my children.

SINGLE PARENTING

Every morning upon rising, I feel as if it's show time. I often joke with friends that a camera crew should follow a single working mom for a day to document how hectic it can be, so the world can get a glimpse of our ups and downs and in-betweens. Some days I miss an appointment, show up late, forget to pack the right items—or worse, lose patience and speak harshly. I apologize to my children. They're generous and forgiving. They even laughed at the time I tried to unlock our front door with our car's key fob and the time I looked all over the school for my keys then discovered I had actually thrown them away with my lunch. Although the job of single parenting seems insurmountable at times, I always make it through to the end of the day. And it's turned out to be easier than the last year of my marriage.

I've faced a paradigm shift when it comes to material items. For example, Hannah and Connor's clothes used to always be name brand, like Gap or Gymboree. As a single parent, I don't have the time or money to care where we get what we need, so I gladly accept the hand-me-down clothes our daycare provider has offered us. This logic has expanded to all of our needs.

SUPPORT SYSTEM

I have an amazing support system now, composed of women and men—true friends who have been there for me in both the happiest and darkest times. My parents have also supported me by accepting Hannah for who she is—not who they want her to be—and nurturing Connor's passion for building with his tools. I discuss my support system in more detail in chapter 11.

FINANCES

Being a single mom of a child with autism has presented a whole other dimension of challenges which affects every decision I make—especially finances. The only thing that gives us a roof over our heads, a dependable vehicle, clothes on our backs, food in our fridge, and extracurricular activities is my paycheck. This sobering reality requires me to perform professionally daily to the best of my ability. There is no room to risk losing my position, because, with the exception of a small amount of child support, I am our only income.

I choose not to have credit card debt because I can't afford the interest, and I don't spend more than I make. To stay on track, I rely on a budget, which organizes funds for weekly and monthly expenses while setting aside a small amount for the kids' college funds and my retirement. These simple steps organize my finances, keep me on track with bill paying, and help me avoid overspending.

SELF-CONFIDENCE

I happen to be a confident person by nature, but I still second-guess myself a lot. If you struggle with feeling insecure and inept, rest in the knowledge you're doing the best you can with the resources you have.

That helps me on the days I waver and question my abilities. Knowing that, I can carry on with some level of confidence even on the emotionally shaky days. The three of us feel like a complete family, and I sit around the dinner table with them while spooning out mashed potatoes and chicken and noodles, thinking how wonderful our lives really are. Connor tells jokes and we all share a giggle, review the day's ups and downs, and pray about current struggles. The Taylor Trio is a blessing—even though just years ago, it felt incomplete. I never imagined it would feel so good to parent solo. I no longer feel as if something is missing. Do I want another man in my life someday? Of course I do, and I know it will happen. But I don't need a man in my life to feel capable and secure as a person and as a parent. Too many people believe in me for me not even to believe in myself. I hope you find that strength in yourself as well. You are capable and should feel confident.

PLAY WITH YOUR KIDS

I'm with my children in the evenings, and I encourage you to be with yours, too. If you're like me, you'll have to consciously choose to be present with them mentally and emotionally. They are our most important use of time. For me, this means if Hannah and Connor are doing homework or playing, I can't be writing, on Facebook, or grading papers. I'm helping with homework, listening to Hannah play piano and violin, allowing them to cook with me, or interacting with them in the SUV while I drive them to activities. When they were little, we'd play Chutes and Ladders and Candyland. Now we play Monopoly, chess, and throw lots of Frisbee. We continue to read individual chapter books together to add to their collections, so that's fun at night. Both of my children have daily devotionals that we also read together. These small acts of connection and attention keep us close so I'm not always task-driven or distracted—and it's a good goal for any parent, whether single or married.

BE CONSISTENT WITH DISCIPLINE

Hannah and Connor know the house rules. I'm firm with discipline, but autism brings on a unique set of behavior challenges where consistency is not always black and white. There's a lot of gray, but I always address behaviors and follow through with consequences. I've found this creates stability in the home and security for the kids—they like knowing what to expect and what they can count on.

TAKE CARE OF YOU

Moms need to refuel. When I attended the Autism Society of America's national conference in Denver, Colorado, in 2015, Cathy Cherry (Certified Autism Specialist and autism parent) said it best: "Sometimes you just have to turn the spotlight off your special one and take a bath." It's okay to be a little selfish.

I enjoy taking walks with friends or just sitting out on the porch while the kids play inside. As a single mom, I don't have a lot of advantages, but I do have a regular opportunity to refuel when the kids are with their father. When I'm alone I like to exercise, write, and watch a couple of my favorite television shows. Even when the kids are at home, they're old enough that I can ask them to stay focused on their games or projects for a few minutes while I sit upstairs and indulge in a new book. When they were younger, I occasionally had someone watch them so I could step away. Remember, taking care of you means you stop thinking about your child's autism, even for only fifteen minutes on a school night. Find a personal outlet. It's not selfish—it's self-preservation. That temporary space makes me a better parent while also encouraging their ability to occupy themselves or successfully play with one another.

ABOLISH GUILT

For a long time, I felt guilty for not raising my children in a two-parent home with more resources and luxuries. But I've witnessed how the kids—and I, too—have learned to enjoy the smaller things, the homemade treats, and the creative activities we dream up together. An ice cream cone after a bike ride in the park is more than enough to satisfy—especially because we're spending more time together on those outings than we did when we purchased the larger, more expensive games and toys and group memberships and store-bought everything like we did in the past. What my children really want is time with their friends and time with me. I need to enjoy this while it lasts. I hope you can, too.

MAINTAIN A DAILY ROUTINE

Hannah's need for structure and routine actually helps our entire family feel calmer and more organized—an unexpected gift of autism. Both of my kids know what to expect when it comes to chores, mealtimes, homework, and bedtime routines. Hannah has a list at the kitchen table, at the garage door, and inside the bathroom cabinet that reminds her to follow various routines in the morning, after school, and before bed. The lists are never to be moved. As the kids have grown older, synching our family calendar on each of their devices for extracurricular activities has also helped them to structure their time and organize necessary items.

I also maintain my own daily routine to stay on top of chores. It varies from day to day, but stays the same from week to week. This routine helps me keep my sanity and ensures no chore is neglected. Following my daily routine, I know when to take out the trash, run the dishwasher, pay the bills that can't be paid online, wash the laundry, and pick up my groceries. Bigger tasks wait for the weekend.

TREAT KIDS LIKE KIDS

Our children only have one childhood, and we can't deny them that. I can see how easy it would be for me as a single parent to try to seek sympathy or companionship from my kids. However, I don't want them to fill that role—they are not responsible for my happiness. Parenting books say not to tell boys they are now the man of the house. I never did this with Connor, but he has said it to me. I allow him to help me "fix" things around the house, but I will never place him in charge of the maintenance of our home.

Solo parenting is full of challenges, but both of my children make me proud that I am blessed with the job of being their mother. So, bring on the dirty laundry, the lawn that needs to be mowed, and the refrigerator that needs to be filled, because there is nothing more important than spending time with both of them.

10 WAYS TO REDUCE SINGLE-PARENT STRESS
- Get a handle on finances.
- Set up a support system.
- Maintain a daily routine.
- Be consistent with discipline.
- Answer questions honestly.
- Treat kids like kids.
- Abolish guilt from your vocabulary.
- Take time for your children.
- Take time for yourself.
- Stay positive.

Wisdom from the Round Table

Lori R.: It's our faith in God that keeps us together. His grace has been sufficient. We are truly each other's best friends, and it's a team effort. We've always had good communication, so if I was struggling or feeling overwhelmed, I would express that to Steve and he would do the same. When one of us was weak, the other became the strong, and vice versa. I wasn't working when Cameron was diagnosed, which was a blessing. When Steve came home, he knew I needed a break because I was the one going to Riley Children's Hospital and therapy three times a week, taking the other three children with me most of the time.

We also learned that you have to ask for help. Our family was six hours away, so that wasn't an option, but we had friends from church we could call on. We also learned not to neglect our marriage. We tried to make date nights or just spend time together after the kids went to bed. We feel like we've weathered the worst of it and are stronger and more compassionate because of it.

Jen: As with any marriage, communication, especially for parents with special needs children, is key. We've also spent a lot of time in prayer and communicate our feelings with one another.

Lori V.: As the mother, don't lose your identity in all of this. My husband left, and I struggled because I had nothing to fall back on.

Susan: My husband, Bruce, has played a huge role in helping to care for Tyler. I couldn't have done it without him. Tyler is six feet two inches tall and weighs two hundred and sixty pounds. Before placed into a residential home, he became aggressive with me. It's humbling to see your husband pull your child off you and then hold him against a wall to keep him from coming after you. That's when we couldn't keep him at home anymore.

Karen: My husband, Bill, and I have always communicated openly with one another about Eric and John's successes and challenges. Our judgments always lie pretty much along the same line with one another. I've always been able to stay at home with the boys. This has been beneficial for our family.

Sarah: My husband and I are blessed that we have family in town to help us care for our kids. I've gone to working part-time in order to eliminate some of the stress. We also have date nights and week-end getaways to focus on just one another. We talk a lot and give one another permission to be truthful—even if it brings pain. There are also times when we know that we need to allow the other space.

CHAPTER TEN

both sides of the table

Meeting Students' Educational Needs

If we can't see a child with autism as capable, interesting, and valuable, no amount of education or therapy we layer on top is going to matter.

—Ellen Notbohm

February 2013
I arrive at school at 8:15, much later than I wanted to arrive. When I dropped the kids off at daycare, Hannah noticed she had forgotten her lunch box and panicked. I had to swing back home to retrieve it—not sure why she hadn't checked her list tacked to the laundry room wall before getting into the car. Now, I punch my security code into the side door of my school and see my teaching colleague and friend, Lori, already waiting for me in the hallway holding a pen, notepad, and file folder. Once again we'll function as a team to advocate for one of our students we believe (really, know) to be on the spectrum—never diagnosed.

As we enter our school's conference room we see that Keegan's parents are already seated. The awkward silence before these meetings begin always disturbs me. Although I've never met Keegan's father, it's fascinating to see how much they resemble one another—amber, straw-textured hair; thin, almost gaunt, body; deep brown eyes; and freckles that seem to align the cheekbones. He appears reticent, like someone who's been told he should be present but doesn't want to be. Keegan's mom's body language speaks a whole different story. She shuffles the papers in front of her, adjusts her glasses, digs around in her bag on the floor, and places a picture of Keegan in the middle of the table. She's the one we've conferenced with several times. She's the one who sent us the list at the beginning of the school year detailing strategies that enable her son to function in the classroom. She's the one who types lengthy emails concerning Keegan's inability to focus on homework in the evenings. In other words, she's already his champion and soon to be his unofficial caseworker.

Procedural safeguards are offered to Keegan's parents, and we all initial our intentioned participation at Keegan's case conference. The lead sixth grade special education teacher distributes copies of Keegan's Multidisciplinary Evaluation Team (MET) report to every member— parents, assistant principal, teachers, school psychologist, educational diagnostician, speech and language pathologist, occupational therapist, and the autism consultant. The answer to our question since August will soon be answered in this substantial collection of closely scrutinized and evaluated data.

While the special education teacher begins by gently citing the reason for Keegan's evaluation along with his background information, I am focused on one thing and one thing only: Did Keegan meet the scoring thresholds to be classified as a student with autism spectrum disorder? *I hastily comb page after page of history, previous assessments, behavioral observations, achievement assessments, behavioral assessments, adaptive behavioral assessments, autism diagnostic observation assessments, language evaluations, and social emotional evaluations. It has to be here somewhere! I feel Lori's eyes heavy on me as she beckons for an answer.*

Finally! I find our answer on page 17. Keegan met the scoring criteria and will be classified as a student with autism spectrum disorder.

The special education teacher continues, and I place the packet back on the table and inconspicuously gesture yes *to Lori.*

Keegan's committee members will also determine his placement and programming today. He'll get the help he needs with a structured Individualized Education Plan. All of our anecdotal notes, meetings, and completed questionnaires advocated an awareness of his tremendous need for support. While Keegan's diagnosis will weigh on his parents, they'll have an answer to so many unanswered behaviors—autism.

An hour later, it's clear. Everyone agrees. The professionals have recognized what the data has already confirmed. The meeting is wrapping up and I'm watching Keegan's mom. Her demeanor is much less anxious than before. I know why. I would say that the three of us got what we wanted, but that would be misinterpreted. Who wants an autism diagnosis? *No, Keegan's mom realizes as she smiles and slips the picture frame into her big quilted tote bag that her son is* different. *There's a reason for his extreme challenges. And now—finally—she has help and a plan—a bittersweet moment indeed.*

THE TABLE METAPHOR

I'm in a unique situation. I'm a regular education teacher who holds special education licensure, and I'm the mom of a daughter that has autism. In terms of autism experience in education, I believe that's a trifecta.

In case conferences, school personnel tend to sit on one side of the table and the student's parents usually sit on the other side of the table. In our school's conference room, parents are always seated on the side directly across from the wall with the screen that displays the document that is also in front of us. For over a decade I only sat on the side with the school personnel. I never thought about the contrast between the two sides until attending Hannah's first developmental preschool case conference at age three. That's when I realized the difference between the two sides of the table that look so similar, but feel so very different.

As teachers, it's our job to discuss a child's strengths and weaknesses, provide classroom observations, share concerns, evaluate the effectiveness of current accommodations and modifications while suggesting others, and help set specific, relevant, attainable goals that can be individually measured. We also ask parents about behaviors and actions that are concerns at home. Many times parents see a different child at home than what we see at school. This often pertains to Hannah. Children with autism work really hard during the day to participate in a world that's often uncomfortable for them. Sometimes they do well at holding it together. It's in the evenings, when they're home and feel safe, that they release all the pent-up anxiety. Children melt down in front of their parents because they know we'll pick up the pieces and love them unconditionally—a blessing and a curse, I guess. I know this all too well from both sides of the table.

As parents, the table is intimidating. The school personnel outnumber parents. In reality, special education law requires that people with different areas of expertise attend—not because they're trying to intimidate you. Just think, everyone around the table has a skill set that can benefit our children; however, it's hard not to feel like you're about to be interrogated by a line of authority figures when seated on the parents' side. It's quiet and awkward at first; anxiety builds in the parents because we don't know what the shool personnel are going to say about our child. Then those lined-up professionals across from us start tossing out specialized vocabulary like executive functioning, social pragmatics, echolalia, stimming, joint attention, affinities, and more. Educators are around this terminology so often that they forget that many parents have no idea what the words mean. The lingo leaves us feeling less capable of helping our child, or worse, as if we're inferior. On that lonely side of the table, as parents we have to sit and hear about behaviors the educators have witnessed and realize our child is doing things we haven't been able to squelch at home, or things we've allowed to continue at home because we weren't aware of how the behaviors make our child look different.

I've felt the strangeness of both sides, and I want to remind you that even though there are different sides of the table, we're all still sitting around *the same table*. The parent and the school are equal partners on the case conference committee and both share decision-making authority. This team effort should be thought of as global in nature—parents know the whole child, and professionals bring wonderful things to the table. As an educator, I can promise you we're all on the child's team— and should be! We're rooting for your child's success and are prepared to work hard to offer the support she needs. And as a parent, I can assure you I know it feels disparaging, but you must advocate for your child while believing no one is trying to intimidate you. Remember that as a parent, you know your child's needs and strengths best. The case conference committee is required to consider your concerns. Your input is valuable and you are an important member of the team! It is all of our jobs—parents and school personnel alike—to work together harmoniously so our children attain the goals cited in their IEP.

I am a staunch advocate in each of my student's case conferences— just as I am in Hannah's when I'm at the table as her mom. I have a genuine concern and respect for everyone gathered around the table and a dedication to the child's best possible outcome. And I don't take for granted the difference one individual can make in a child's life. I believe my system permits me to be so vocal in conferences because of my age, my teaching experience, my education, my experience with Hannah, and my endless search for tools and instructional strategies to make every one of my students the best they can be. School systems understand the need for at least one seasoned professional to be seated at the table, so you'll see who has this kind of freedom and offers key input when you're at the table.

I'm also there for the parents. They need explanations, information, and hope. In a conference not long ago, a parent was sad that her child never wanted to have friends over to the house. Her child was never asked to others' homes, either, and she said he didn't even understand how sad this should make him feel. That's when I stepped in to say that what makes parents happy isn't necessarily what makes our child happy. In other words, our happy is not theirs. All we want is our child's happiness, right? That should be enough. If that means just hanging out with the family in the evenings and on weekends, so be it. It's rewarding for me to be a novel resource for parents. Hopefully someone will offer you that kind of input and support; if not, that's okay. Don't expect it. After all, not every educator happens to also have a child with autism! Find that level of understanding and insight through an outside support group.

CHOOSE YOUR CHILD'S SCHOOL SYSTEM

The school district we live in now is not the school district we lived in before Hannah's autism diagnosis. As you may recall, we moved closer to where we worked so Hannah and I could be home in time for her in-home therapies and my husband wouldn't have quite the commute to work. We would later discover that our new district came highly recommended by others I would meet in the autism community.

In her book *The Way I See It*, Temple Grandin explains how parents often ask her opinion if they should change schools. She has a simple way to help a parent decide. "Ask this question: Is your child making progress and improving where he is now?" She advises the parents to keep the child where he is if the answer is yes, because they can always look into supplementing with extracurricular programs and therapies. If the answer is no, the child is not improving or making progress, take a look at the school's limitations. Wasting precious time and energy fighting the school to try to get it to change doesn't help the child. Because that's the end goal, she says, "giving the child as much opportunity to learn and acquire needed skills in as supportive an environment as possible." If you don't have it, move to find it.[21] Also remember that a combative attitude doesn't help to make progress with the school. Your relationship should be an alliance—not an adversarial face-off.

When you choose your school, you're choosing your teacher. And the teacher has a pivotal role in your child's life. Highly regarded educator and author Haim Ginott said it well: "I've come to a frightening conclusion that I am the decisive element in the classroom."[22] He's right! It's the teacher who will have your child in their classroom for ten months or possibly more for six hours a day. Due to that long-term impact, I suggest you find out by either asking the teacher or the administration:

Does your child's teacher(s) have experience teaching children with autism? Prior experience with children on the spectrum helps deliver faster interventions and appropriate behavior modifications. There's a huge learning curve, and what works for one child may not work for another. Experience is the best teacher.

Do they have special education licensure? It is absolutely necessary that your child's Teacher of Record (TOR) have a special education license; however, if your child is mainstreamed into the general education classroom, there's only a small chance that those teachers will have special education licensure.

What is the class size and ratio of students to teachers and assistants, and what evidence-based teaching practices are utilized? The class size and ratio of students to teachers and assistants needs to be directly related to the functioning level, medical needs, and behavior concerns of those students in the class. There are a number of successful evidence-based teaching practices available for educators. The question is if the teaching practices the school uses are compatible with your child's learning style.

How do the nonverbal students communicate? In today's schools, assistive technologies, augmentative communication, and visual supports can foster speech development. Examples include devices and apps with pictures that your child touches to produce words. On a simpler level, visual supports can include pictures and groups of pictures that your child can use to indicate requests and thoughts.

How are therapy services provided? All services including OT, PT, and ST should be provided during the school day by a licensed therapist.

Does the school system have an autism consultant or coordinator? An autism consultant or coordinator is a beneficial resource for parents and teachers. Because the autism consultant doesn't teach classes, they have time available during the day to observe students and in-service teachers and meet with parents. Some of them even run social groups.

How does the staff handle behavior issues? Challenging behavior must be handled immediately or the behavior will become increasingly intense. Physical and mental health concerns must be addressed first. Staff must determine why this behavior is happening. Then behavioral and educational supports should be used to teach replacement skills/ behaviors and self-regulation. Lastly, a behavior plan must be put into place and reviewed as needed.

PARENTAL RIGHTS

Parents must understand the basic caveats of special education law. I use www.specialeducationguide.com and www.wrightslaw.com as resources.

Hannah was able to start intervention services at the early age of sixteen months only because our pediatrician made me aware of the services. Prior to that visit with the pediatrician, I didn't know the services were available. If your child is under three, these early inter-vention services are provided in-home and are the way to go. But please remember that your child must first be evaluated and qualify.

When your child turns three, he can be reevaluated or evaluated for the first time for entry into your local developmental preschool. Devel-opmental preschools offer help with daily skills, occupational therapy, speech therapy, and physical therapy. Hannah attended developmental preschool a little over two years, and our school system even provided transportation. What I appreciated the most from the developmental preschool staff was their help with Hannah's everyday skills, like eat-ing, teeth brushing, and toilet training.

The Individuals with Disabilities Education Act (IDEA) is a fed-eral law that requires schools to serve the educational needs of eligible students with disabilities. Schools must evaluate students suspected of having a disability; however, not every child with learning and atten-tion issues qualifies for special education services under IDEA. Parents can request an evaluation if they see concerns. IDEA ensures that students with disabilities have access to a free and appropriate public education (FAPE). Parents have the right to participate in all meetings regarding evaluation and placement—in fact, both evaluation and placement require parental consent. Schools must provide the education in the least restrictive environment (LRE), which means schools must teach students with disabilities in the general education classroom whenever possible. It's important to remember that special education is a service—not a space. Procedural safeguards give parents rights and protections. Your child's IEP must be followed—as law clearly states. Make sure social goals are also written into your child's IEP. If you have concerns, please follow the chain of command, starting with your child's teacher. Parents also have the right to challenge educational decisions through due process procedures. IDEA covers kids from infancy through high school graduation or age twenty-one (whichever comes first). Be sure that your child's weaknesses are supported, strengths recognized, and abilities encouraged.

Parents are sometimes concerned about the amount of time their child may or may not spend in the general education setting. First of all, from an educator's perspective, I can tell you I've seen benefits to having exposure with same-aged peers who are modeling appropriate language, gestures, skills, and abilities. However, the bigger question is if the child can keep up with the pace and rigor of the grade-level curriculum with accommodations. Can the child work at grade level with supports? If not, the school can look for situations in which inclusion or mainstreaming may also be possible, like physical education, music, and art classes, as well as lunch and recess. Also keep in mind, although some individuals use the words mainstreaming and inclusion interchangeably, they actually have two different premises. The concept of **mainstreaming** is based on the fact that a student with disabilities may benefit from being in a general education classroom, both academically and socially. The concept of **inclusion** is based on the idea that students with disabilities should not be segregated, but should be included in a classroom with their typically developing peers. Proponents of inclusion tend to put more of an emphasis on life preparation and social skills than on the acquisition of level-appropriate academic skills.

Sometimes children are academically able to succeed, but their emotional maturity is years behind, so when they're mainstreamed or in an inclusion class they feel out of place with peers pursuing completely different interests. This can often lead to feelings of isolation and loneliness. As a parent, I watched Hannah struggle at the beginning of fifth grade to connect with girls in her classroom. They would talk nonstop about music and social media while Hannah was still stuck on cats, cats, and more cats. She felt out of step and out of place. I talked with Hannah about the benefits of being more *interested* than *interesting*, but at that age she said that it just merely felt like acting. And we all know that acting like someone we're not is worse than being miserable. In his book, *Be Different*, John Elder Robison states, "You should respond to what others say, not just speak what's on your mind." I believe that was great advice for Hannah.

Over time, she thankfully did find a niche of kids that adored cats, still loved My Little Pony, and were hooked on the *Warriors* book series. Then, with the help of her behavioral specialist, she was able to stretch to successfully connect with others. However, the interim was painful for us both. The school can and should always work closely with the parent to determine the best approach for the individual child.

CASE CONFERENCES AND INDIVIDUAL EDUCATION PLANS

Individual Education Plans (IEPs) are generally reviewed once a year, and this meeting is referred to as the annual case review (ACR). No matter which side of the table I'm representing at a case conference, I always bring a list of questions that I want answered. The meeting is not over until each one of my questions is crossed off. Make your own list of questions as the parent and bring it along to the ACR. Don't be afraid to get answers.

I not only ask a lot of questions during conferences, but I also take copious notes at each one, my pen flying across the page. With the multitude of professionals gathered around the table, I learn several new things at each conference and I'm not afraid to jot down a quick note to email the professional about later. Hannah's behavioral therapist,

Kait, blew me away at Hannah's last conference using exceptional terminology that was new to me. I jotted down terms like "errorless teaching" and "echoicly."

You might ask if there's a home base in the school where a child can retreat if she becomes agitated, upset, or dysregulated. At our school, many children benefit from sensory breaks either seated in a beanbag chair or on a therapy ball, covered with a weighted blanket or wearing a weighted vest, or manipulating fidget toys, Wikki Stix, or putty. Given my unusual perspective from sitting on both sides of the table, I've been able to make recommendations like this at my school and other local children's venues, but if I were only a parent and not also a teacher, I would meet with someone and ask anyway.

Case conferences are not a time to get sidetracked and compare your special needs child to their siblings or entertain topics that are not pertinent to your child's IEP. The committee understands that your child's challenges aren't a reflection of your parenting. And hearing that your child isn't good in math because you were never good in math sounds like an excuse. Chances are, while those teachers are sitting in the conference, someone else is teaching their classes. Time is precious and so is your child—stay focused to understand the situation thoroughly and get her what she needs.

A SUCCESSFUL PARTNERSHIP BETWEEN SCHOOL AND HOME

A successful relationship between parents and teachers will provide powerful underpinning for your child as she transitions from home to school and back again each day. You must both communicate and help one another out. Teachers can reinforce the life skills and independence that parents are working on at home. Likewise, parents can help teachers by reviewing specific academic skills that their children are having trouble with in school. Start the year off right by implementing the suggestions listed in the text box. Also, this isn't your responsibility, but make certain your child's teacher has their current IEP. I'm also always upfront with Hannah's teachers at the very beginning of the year. I share strengths as well as areas in which she struggles in school, which is mostly independence, executive functioning skills, and social pragmatics.

When Hannah was younger, a log book would travel back and forth between home and school, and everyone who had worked with Hannah each day—from the teacher and therapist to the counselor and autism specialist—would write a little note explaining what they worked on, skills that needed to be reinforced at home, successes, or concerns. As Hannah aged we stopped the log book and wrote notes back and forth in her agenda only when we had something we needed to tell the other one. I want teachers to be totally honest with me. I don't want them to dismiss Hannah's inappropriate behaviors or struggles. If I don't know about them, I can't do my part to help her with them. Hannah's agenda was initialed every day by her teacher to make sure she had written down the evening's assignments. If your child's teacher or autism specialist doesn't recommend a system like this, feel free to ask for something that works for the both of you. I made sure this was written into Hannah's IEP during elementary school. Now that Hannah is going into the seventh grade, I expect the teachers and I will handle most communication via email with an occasional phone call and/or meeting.

SIX TIPS FOR A SMOOTHER BACK-TO-SCHOOL EXPERIENCE

- Create a personalized story or picture schedule for your child's school day. Contact your child's school to access his daily schedule. A picture of your child's teacher and classroom may also be helpful.
- Promote communication between previous teachers and your child's new teacher. The teacher should share teaching techniques and behavior strategies that worked well. If your child attends specific therapies during the day, have those specialists talk with your child's teacher as well.
- Make sure all of your child's medical information is up to date with the school. If any medications have

changed during the summer, make sure the school notes the change. Inform the teacher of any allergies.

* Keep in mind that although you need to advocate for what is best for your child, you also need to work cooperatively with the school. Review your child's IEP and make contact with the new teacher—introduce yourself and touch upon the most important points of your child's disability. Do not assume teachers already have all of this information. Be honest and open with the teacher. He or she has the same goals for your child as you do.

* Volunteer your time making materials, being an extra hand, or helping with special projects and events. This is a valuable way to observe how the classroom operates. And by eliminating some of the teacher's busywork, the teacher will have more time with the children, including yours.

* If your child is a bus rider, find out if the bus driver, bus number, and pick-up and drop-off times are the same as the previous year. If the driver has changed, contact the new driver to discuss any concerns.

EXPECTING SCHOOLS TO FIX OUR CHILDREN

While discussing this chapter with the Round Table, Lori R. shared some wisdom that was particularly valid. She said:

"It has been my experience that a lot of parents want the school system to *fix* their child. When that doesn't happen as expected, then they believe it's the school system's fault. I feel like I have a strong faith, but I'm also a realist. Parents cannot be unrealistic in their expectations about what a school system has funding for. We could've gone to court and demanded the school system pay for Cameron's ABA therapy. But because we chose to work with, not against, the school system, we came up with a plan within the means of the school system that was a good fit for everyone.

"As a parent, you have to do your homework and know what works best for your child. When you approach educators with the attitude that this is a team effort, and that you are open to suggestions and willing to try new things, I think that your relationship with the school system is so much better and makes them more open and want to listen to the parent. Pick your battles."

VALUABLE TEACHING TRUISMS

Autism expert Dr. Ivar Lovaas said, "If they can't learn the way we teach, we teach the way they learn."[23] Teachers must be open to differentiating the delivery of their subject area's content in a variety of ways. Of the numerous teaching resources that discuss best practices to use for our students on the spectrum, my favorite is Ellen Notbohm's *Ten Things Your Student With Autism Wishes You Knew.* In her book she states, "Because I think differently, my autism requires that you teach differently. In order to teach me to color inside the lines, you may have to reach outside those lines. To get me to see life and learning as a palette of colors, you have to start by understanding that through my eyes, life's experiences are black and white, all or nothing."[24] I've seen that "black and white, all or nothing" in Hannah at home and in the classroom. A related bit of insight is that fair doesn't look the same for everyone, and our school system seems to have made this normal and accepted. I've never been questioned by a student or a parent why some students have different assignments or classroom work than the rest. I believe that differentiation has been an accepted philosophy in our school system for so long now that kids don't even pay attention. I see one student's accommodations the same as another student's eyeglasses. Both students should get what they need to succeed. No one would take away a student's eyeglasses, so why not provide accommodations?

I use several strategies in my classroom geared for students on the spectrum that benefit all learners. When I'm working with a student on life skills, for example, and they're having trouble learning by watching others, I use personalized stories. I've had our school system's autism consultant create personalized stories in which a protagonist (often named Hannah) must practice skills such as how to transition success-fully between classes, find a friend at recess, and pack up for the bus. They're geared for special needs students, but the entire classroom can listen and learn from them. If the story has been individualized for a student, I would never share it with the entire class, but stories present-ing general principles are good for teaching organizational skills, social pragmatics, and self-care. In situations involving group work, I either assign roles within the group, set the structure of the group as divide and conquer, assign peer buddies to prompt the students with autism, or, if they prefer, sometimes I even allow the students with autism to work by themselves.

I also try to use procedures in my classroom that allow our class-room to flow more efficiently. When giving directions to the class, I'll ask my students to repeat the directions back to me. I also speak slower and allow for wait time for their individual motor processing when asking a question. Each child has a different speed—even students who aren't on the spectrum may need more time to process what I've said. Teachers must remember that students with autism are motor plan-ning by receiving and deciphering meaning from the question, while also planning an answer and tapping into expressive language to put the words together in a meaningful way. That's a lot to manage. Before Hannah's language greatly improved, I'd ask her a question and go on about my household work—forgetting that I'd asked her a ques-tion. After a few minutes would pass, she'd yell out the answer. In the movie *Rain Man*, Tom Cruise says this about Dustin Hoffman's char-acter with autism, "He is answering a question from a half hour ago."

There are many ways in which I create an environment in my class-room that values efficiency and helping one another out. As Hannah's sixth grade math and science teacher, I was privy to interactions every day when other students helped my daughter be more efficient. For in-stance, her friends often gave her prompts in class like, *clear off your desk, get out your laptop,* or *write down your assignment.* If she was having a difficult time understanding a math problem presented on the board, another student in her group would explain it to her in a different way. I'm also a stickler for finding an appropriate organiza-tional tool that works for student, teacher, and parent. Everyone must buy into the plan and know the system. Finally, if a student's behavior is a distraction to either themselves or other students, there must be a behavior plan in place. I know as both a parent and an educator that behavior is a symptom of discomfort, so I look for and find the triggers (discomforts) that are causing the symptoms. Work with the school in determining what triggers could be adversely affecting your child in the school environment. Behavior plans should also be constantly re-evaluated based on efficacy.

Time is an important executive functioning skill. Many students on the spectrum don't move with any sense of urgency. Prompting these students to pack up early allows for more successful transitions. Coats and lunch boxes must be stored in one specific place or they will be lost. Hannah and many other students with autism I've taught over the years will have multiple lunch boxes all over the place and claim they have no idea where they are, but everyone else in the class knows (it's hard to miss her cat lunch boxes).

Students with autism will draw, rock in their seats, bounce on their seats, play with the lead in their mechanical pencils, design origami, and line up every marker in their materials box if they aren't given some type of fidget tool. You may want to supply your child with his own fidget tool if the school doesn't provide one, and check with the teacher to help her understand how it will help. You might even gently suggest a few rules that your child understands and will honor and promise to reinforce those same rules in the home.

Most students on the spectrum have a particular interest or hobby. Feel free to communicate these to the teacher and encourage her to watch for more. At home and at school, you'll enter your child's world and help him learn more and more. I can't tell you the number of topics I've explored in order to relate to my students on the spectrum: anime, robotics, *Dr. Who*, *Star Wars*, chess, Minecraft, and more. Then I was able to relate to other students with the same passions (special needs or not). Any teacher with autism experience knows how important this doorway can be. Share this information with your child's teacher! When teachers use this doorway, kids also feel valued and respected. They will no longer be a student who needs intermittent redirection.

KIDS ON THE SPECTRUM IN THE CLASSROOM (AND A FEW BLUNDERS)

My experience in the classroom with students on the spectrum has helped me understand the way autism affects one's view of a situation. My students with autism are challenging and amazing at the same time. Earlier in my career, I quickly learned that I needed to be as direct as possible when communicating with students with autism. One year I asked the class, "Did that information just go in one ear and out the other?" A young man with autism responded, "Can information really just go straight into one ear and then just go out the other?"

On another day I said, "I'm so sorry it's time for my class to be over. I know you really dislike having to go to Mr. Bevel's class right now, but you really have to." That same boy came up to my desk when I released the class and told me it's not nice to talk about others like that, especially nice people like Mr. Bevel.

Not too long ago, I thought I was captivating my entire science class with the legendary story of Sir Isaac Newton's discovery of the law of universal gravitation. I had just dropped my foam apple on a student's head and was right at the point where Newton asks about the force that keeps the moon revolving around Earth when a student with Asperger's syndrome asked me how long I was going to drone on and on with that inaccurate story? I had no comeback—at all.

Another student enjoyed origami during class and lined up his markers according to the light spectrum on his desk. He was inhibited to do grade-level math but could solve higher level algebra problems in his head. This student also rocked in his chair and had the precision of a diamond cutter when attacking his "going home" routine. He packed his materials the same exact way every single day.

Several years ago I had another student with Asperger's syndrome who was very quiet in class but was a brilliant writer—no doubt gifted. He used a huge voice in his science fiction stories. I asked him where he found the words to write so vividly? His answer would be the same one Hannah would use eight years later. He said, "I look in the thought bubble above my head."

A WORD CONCERNING
MY PASSION FOR TEACHING

Although this book is about our family's journey with autism in order to help others, I feel it's also important to share a piece of my identity that was not lost over the last decade. Teaching has always been, and will always be, a constant in my life. My passion for teaching sixth graders is at the core of my being and fills me with great pride every day.

My students (with and without autism), along with their parents, have supported me enthusiastically in all of my pursuits outside of the classroom, including autism awareness walks, speaking events, and creative pursuits. Their encouragement has been astounding!

If you have a similar passion, hold onto it. Don't allow autism to deprive you of all the activities you love—especially those that form your core identity.

TEN THINGS YOUR CHILD'S TEACHER
NEEDS TO KNOW

- Current medications and allergies
- Useful motivational techniques
- Sensory challenges
- Dietary/toiletry/health needs
- Most significant strengths and weaknesses
- Possible triggers
- Language barriers
- Prior successful learning tools (Time Timer, fidgets, weighted vest, sensory breaks, visual schedule, communication device, and more)
- Best method of communication for parents
- Affinities, interests, and passions
- Prior successful teaching methodologies

⚘ **Wisdom from the Round Table** ⚘

Lori R.: When Cameron was first diagnosed and entered developmental preschool, he had teachers who had no experience working with children on the spectrum. His therapists at the time also worked in the district we're in now and discreetly told us we needed to move. I then observed classrooms in the new system and met with the Director of Special Education. I was impressed, and they made me feel as if I had the most important voice in his education plan.

Cameron had a one-on-one assistant until his second year in high school when he was more independent. His IEP had been followed to the letter. The high school also has excellent programs to offer students like Cameron.

Jen: I really didn't allow myself to process the fact that Noah was different until spring of his seventh grade year. Signing my name to a form that would place him on a resource education track for the rest of his school years was very, very difficult. Noah wouldn't be able to earn a Core 40 diploma or take many classes with his elementary school friends.

Lori V.: At the beginning of sixth grade, the district hired an autism consultant that became Byron's advocate and mentor from that point on until his graduation. She was by far Byron's lifeline in school and for social activities. She understood Byron completely and was his voice. She helped teach him how to tell the difference between friends and those who use you for humor or bullying and to cope better and accept that he will always feel differently and that's okay. Byron still talks of her today and misses her.

Susan: Before Tyler turned twenty-one, I felt I knew his daily routine and was more aware of his successes and challenges. However, now that he's in a residential home, some of that insight has vanished. I'm still not sure how I feel about that.

Karen: Both Eric and John were truly blessed to have so many caring and wonderful teachers. They were able to look beyond my boys' challenges and build upon their strengths. I credit Eric's third grade teacher the most. She was well trained, recognized his autistic characteristics, helped with the diagnosis, and made an enormous impact with both of my boys.

Sarah: Mitchell's Teachers of Record (TOR) have always helped to carry out accommodations and modifications in the classroom as stated in his IEP. Now that he's in high school, he's receiving less services (pull-out), but getting more direction in self-advocacy and organizational skills. These caveats are essential to Mitchell's continued success.

CHAPTER ELEVEN
find your warriors

Friendship isn't about who you've known the longest. It's about who walked into your life and said, "I'm here for you," and proved it.

—Unknown

May 2015

Today is the fourth grade talent show at Hannah's school. I found out about the talent show the day before tryouts. Hannah ran off of the bus that day, found me in the house, and stuck the permission slip, dated one week prior, into my hands. With a demanding and anxious tone that matched the look on her face, she ordered, "Mom. Talent show tryouts are tomorrow, and you have to help me with this! I want to sing Meghan Trainor's 'Lips Are Movin' in front of the entire fourth grade."

Hannah probably knew she was going to try out for the show ever since it was announced but never organized a plan to help make that happen—one of her deficits. Far be it from me to get in the way of something my daughter so adamantly wants to accomplish, though, so we downloaded the instrumental version on iTunes, printed the lyrics, and looked in her closet for something fashionable to wear.

Hannah had recently performed as Mrs. Potts in her school's production of Beauty and the Beast. *She liked carrying a solo tune while performing front and center for her peers. She was yearning for more.*

Results were posted the next day, and Hannah would indeed get to perform again. With her incredible memory, she quickly memorized the song's lyrics. "Will you be able to attend?" she asked me. Of course I would try my hardest to find coverage for my class, but any day in May is challenging.

Now, the day of the talent show, I scurry around to find an aide to cover my class. No luck. My teaching partner, Lori, says we can place all sixty students into her room, but I don't want my problem to create more work and a change in plans for her. Hannah's elementary school is only five minutes away. I text my friend, Deb, who teaches the fourth grade—the same grade as Hannah—and she's quick to reach Hannah.

As I speak with Hannah on the phone, I detect her anxiety. "You'll do a phenomenal job," I assure her, "but I may not be able to make it." Silence. She's disappointed. I feel for the first time that I'm not putting my family first, but I have thirty kids in my classroom right now. Guilt overtakes me.

What if she forgets a word and has a meltdown? What if the music doesn't work, and she's aggravated beyond control? What if she just needs her mother for confidence? Or, worse than anything, what if her audience of peers laugh at her? I feel as if I'm the only one in the world that has the ability to calm her emotions.

By the time Hannah hands the phone to Deb, I resolve to have my teaching partner take all sixty kids. I tell Deb to text me ten minutes before Hannah is on stage, and that'll be my cue to leave. I'll get there in no time. Deb decides not to tell Hannah in case my intention fails, but what could go wrong?

I receive Deb's text at 2:30.

I've already prepared my students, so they quickly move next door. My car rolls out of the parking lot at 2:33, and that's when I see it— the train! Trains don't run on an exact schedule through my town, so why does it choose this minute to run? I scan to my right—the end is nowhere in sight. I text Deb, begging her to stall, and she has Hannah moved to the last act of her grade level. At 2:45 I consider an alternate route, but there probably isn't time. Where is the end of this train? After a graffiti-covered, yellow boxcar passes I get Deb's last text, "She's going on. I'm videoing. She'll do great. She's got this!"

Upon arriving at her school, I run straight to the gym at 2:50, bypassing the office staff with a frantic wave. I enter the gym, and I see Hannah standing beside the bleachers. She gives me the biggest hug ever, and she hands me Deb's iPad. She says, "Mom, let's go out into the hallway and you can watch me. Deb recorded it for you and told me you'd watch it as soon as you got here."

She had done it. No meltdown. In fact, she beamed with pride. Another crisis averted. And this daughter of mine is no longer the fragile, dependent child I had to coax out of the stands to shoot a basketball. She's gaining confidence each day. This girl is emerging.

Hannah, Connor, and I have a tribe of good people, like Deb and Lori, who are there for each of us when I can't do it all on my own. My warriors have helped me survive tumultuous storms that have raged out of my control. They gave me strength when I lost the life I thought I couldn't live without. They assured me I was beautiful, lovely, and loved just the way I was. They taught me that a person does not have to do it all alone, and there's no shame in asking for help. Although I tried to hide it, they knew when I was running on fumes, in need of fuel to keep going. And they supplied it. No one can do autism alone. Our warriors are necessary for our survival.

I'll never forget Deb running across the school's parking lot to catch me before my appointment with the guardian ad litem. You may recall that in chapter 9 I discussed the need to be interviewed by a court-appointed GAL to finalize custody arrangements. I was going for the interview after teaching one day, and Deb's school dismissed about the same time as mine. She had arrived at my school and gone in only to find that I had already been picked up by another friend. She went outside, saw our vehicle, and ran across the parking lot trying to wave us down. The hug and good wishes were worth her efforts.

And my friends continued to show up. While teaching summer school, I received a call from the YMCA's supervisor saying my kids were dropped off by their dad without a lunch. I didn't even know that the YMCA had ever watched them. Why weren't they with their dad? I couldn't leave my class, so my friend Lori ran to the grocery, bought their favorites, and delivered them for me. After I disclosed to my friend Cindy that Hannah had autism and I was expecting Connor, she prayed with me. My principal announced my Teacher of the Year award during the most grueling time in my life.

I hate to admit this, but until Hannah's diagnosis and my divorce, I'm not sure I truly believed in how good people are—I'm not sure I trusted their authenticity. When I was hit with hard times, I ran to those I really loved and they blew me away with how genuine and caring they are. To this day, they provide practical, moral, emotional, and relational support through the entire storm—not just the beginning. Friends and family who understand and accept Hannah don't show us pity or act as if a lack of discipline is the problem—when my patience is maxed, they offer a calm demeanor to help redirect Hannah's emotions. You must also surround yourself with positive people who want the best for you and your family. The best of friends will be there for you without judgment. Most people want to help. Let them.

I do understand that for a variety of reasons some moms may not have had the opportunities for friendships that I had. You might see if people at your workplace will let you lean on them a little more and find you have a coworker who will become closer through the process. Your warriors might be from your family or neighbors who have seen your plight and offered to help. Even medical professionals become part of the tribe, the team that we turn to—not, of course, for something like babysitting or a shoulder to cry on, but to get professional advice about developmental stages and acute needs. We see them so often, doctors and therapists can become some of our warriors.

You'll encounter people who mean well. They'll say things like, "God never gives you more than you can handle." What does that mean? That I have strong enough shoulders to carry all of this myself? I appreciate their faith, but I felt like telling those people, "Hey, I've come to see that I'm pretty strong, but maybe you could ask God to give me a few more people to help carry this heavy load? I'm pretty overwhelmed by myself over here!" While I never said that out loud, I realize now that I ended up with an amazing support system composed of exactly the right people to walk with me and shoulder the load. I had exactly what I joked that I needed, especially in the darkest days, and the three of us wouldn't be where we are today without their help.

FRIENDS

My dear friend for the last twenty-three years, Lori, has been my rock and compass through the last decade. She is beautiful inside and out. She spoke at our wedding, celebrated both Hannah and Connor's arrivals at the hospital, left work when my husband was experiencing heart problems, and sat on the bench behind me in court during my divorce. There is no friend more loyal. I've been blessed to teach sixth grade with her for twenty-three years, and we have co-taught for over eleven.

Lori organized an intervention one morning when my husband and I were ready to separate. She served brunch to my inner circle of friends. Following brunch, they had me sit on the couch. Each friend around the room took their turn to offer advice I needed to get through the next few months and years. Lori has also provided support in my professional life because she's ultra-organized and likes to lead our teaching team. This takes a tremendous amount of pressure off me. When my divorce was final after two long years, Lori planned a trip downtown with all of my friends in hopes of lifting my spirits. It worked! They had me laughing and realizing I was surrounded with joy and strength. In a lovely culmination, Lori has been Hannah's language arts and social studies teacher this past year, reinforcing Hannah's natural love of language and learning and pressing her to explore even more of her interests within those fields of study. Lori has helped me raise my daughter and son and rebuild my life.

Turn to your friends. One warrior often rises above the rest, positioned well to see your needs and round up others to serve you.

FAMILY

My parents live four hours away, but they visit and help out when they can, embracing Hannah for exactly who she is. Her behaviors

have never frustrated them and they don't harbor unrealistic expectations for her. My mother sometimes travels with me as an autism
advocate to various conferences. And, as embarrassing as it felt, my
parents helped me financially with court costs associated with gaining
custody of my children and the preservation of my teaching pension.
If your parents aren't able to step in and help, you might have a sibling who is able to support your needs as a warrior for you and your
child, and don't forget the possibility of extended family like aunts
and uncles.

Not everyone has supportive family, however. All the more reason
to seek out and build a core friendship base and see what other people
can fill in gaps.

MEDICAL SUPPORT

Every once in a while, a compassionate doctor begins to feel like he's
become a friend to your family, but medical professionals cannot and
should not serve the same role as close friends or family. Nevertheless,
they clearly serve a critical role in your lives, fighting for your child.

DOCTORS AND STAFF

I will be forever thankful to Dr. McIntire for suggesting at an early age
that Hannah had a pervasive developmental disorder. He pointed me
in the right direction to get help. Without his early detection, Hannah
would not have had the early window for intervention. During one
visit to his office, Hannah grew agitated as soon as we set foot into
his office, flapping her arms, crying, and screaming. Dr. McIntire just
happened to be speaking to his secretary. We were there for a well
visit, so he asked what had upset her. I said that when I picked her up
from school, I drove a different route to the office than I normally do,
and she was not happy and this behavior would continue throughout
the evening. Dr. McIntire knew that Hannah's school was within five
miles, so he suggested we go back to Hannah's school and drive to
his office by the route she knew. I did that, and the rest of the evening
was peaceful. We need doctors who understand our plight and make

accommodations, because he didn't cancel our appointment—he let us come back ten minutes later.

His office staff always knew that Hannah's appointments needed to be consistent. As busy as they were, Tina and Nikki always made sure Hannah was placed in the room with the barn, as that was Hannah's expectation. Gina, the secretary, always made Hannah feel special, which made me so fond of her. One time I called for a sick visit, and Gina couldn't get us in until the next day. As soon as I told her it was for Hannah, she said, "Why didn't you tell me this was for Hannah? I didn't know who was calling. Of course! You bring my girl in as soon as you can." Dr. McIntire also had a secretary named Sarah who would send Hannah stickers through the mail. She secretly pulled me aside one day and said, "You're doing this alone. You're an amazing mom. I have so much respect for you. I will never forget the day Dr. McIntire suggested a pervasive developmental delay. Hannah is so blessed to have you as her advocate and mom."

THERAPISTS

Hannah had excellent therapists, but the one who made the biggest difference in her life was her First Steps and later her private occupational therapist, Tara. Tara understood how Hannah perceived the world and helped her conquer the sensory challenges that interfered with her progress. She was the most influential force driving Hannah's progress with early intervention. Her skill set, determination, and work ethic helped rewire neurological pathways that impeded Hannah's development. If you can find a warrior like that, especially in the early stages of intervention, you are very fortunate.

CHILDCARE PROVIDERS

Hannah and Connor have also had two wonderful in-home daycare providers who have been there to serve both of my children's needs. Nancy was there in the very beginning with Hannah's diagnosis. She graciously allowed Hannah's evaluators and therapists into her home and worked with them to meet Hannah's needs. Nancy played a huge role in helping with Hannah's dietary needs and digestive challenges. She would make sure Hannah was comfortable getting onto the developmental preschool bus and was there for her at drop-off. Our second daycare providers—Dawn, Dana, and Diana—worked earnestly with Hannah to help her to interact with other children and communicate. They knew the vigilance needed to monitor Hannah's medicine and nutrition. They also did a phenomenal job with Hannah's schedule, juggling three preschools in one year. They even aided with transportation to one of them and transported Connor, too, when it came time. Diana also went to court to testify on my behalf to be awarded custody, and Dawn continues to provide hand-me-downs for Hannah. Both of these providers allowed me to go to work every single day without worry about my children. We were blessed to have them in our lives. Find trusted caregivers you can rely on, who will love your children and learn all they can about autism if they aren't already knowledgeable or certified. These people are warriors for you and your child, so take the time to research quality childcare in your area.

As much as possible, seek support from medical professionals, therapists, and childcare providers who look out for you and your child's needs. They won't replace friends—nor should they—but they are warriors fighting for your success, and the best will understand the unique needs of your child with autism.

GROUP SUPPORT

You'll find warriors in a range of places throughout your community, like your religious affiliation, clubs, and support groups.

CHURCHES AND OTHER FAITH-BASED SUPPORT

The day after my husband told me he was leaving, a dear friend took me to seek counsel from her pastor. Pastor Karen listened, counseled, and prayed for our family. Shortly after, we began attending her church. The congregation surrounded me with peace and love. My children and I still worship there today. Suzanne, a volunteer counselor trained through a denominational program, was assigned to provide prayer and counseling for our family. She listened to my struggles and helped me find strength in prayer. Your faith or religious community may have something similar in place or you might visit a place your friends attend. Ask around.

SUPPORT GROUPS

The church also offered a Single and Parenting Friday night support group. Trained babysitters provided childcare, so there was no excuse not to attend. I decided to go in hopes of giving my dear friends a break. They had patiently listened to me unload my struggles for years—it was time to find a few new listening ears. At my first meeting, a fit, petite, beautiful blonde woman welcomed attendees at the door. I thought, "What could this woman know about working full-time, going through a divorce, raising kids by yourself, and facing daily financial stress?" I soon found out that Kim was the most down-to-earth woman I'd ever met. She proved to be a selfless, helpful, encouraging nurturer, eager to serve every single one of us. Kim listened to each of our stories and never interrupted us. She was empathetic and nonjudgmental. She quickly became one of my best friends.

The support group was good for every member—we learned we were not going through this alone. The program provided guidance in many areas: finances, parenting, balancing life's responsibilities, religious education, and grieving divorce. We could relate to one another's difficulties. Look for support groups like this. Mine was faith-based and geared to single people. You might find an autism support group where a fellow attendee offers more than you ever expected. Or perhaps a civic group you're already part of can supply you with that kind of empathetic, nonjudgmental friendship.

NEIGHBORS AND SCHOOL FRIENDS

I am humbled to now think of the people I can call at any time and know for certain they would drop everything to help us, especially in my core friendship base, but I learned another layer of friends have been there all along—I just never asked them for help.

NEIGHBORS

Two of our neighbors include us in all of their gatherings, help me maintain my home and yard, ensure I'm not by myself for holidays, share their amazing desserts including cranberry bars and hummingbird cake, and are only a house away on each side. I've awakened to a foot of snow and heard a neighbor moving it off my driveway with his snow blower. My neighbors save me when I'm in tears and about ready to throw in the towel on my lawnmower, totally puzzled on how to raise Connor's bike seat, or have to resort to turning the water off to the toilet because it just keeps running. Because our family isn't keen on watching television, they've also been known to knock on our patio door to alert us to upcoming severe weather so we can seek shelter in their basements.

WORK FRIENDS AND MY CHILDREN'S FRIENDS' PARENTS

The teachers I've taught with are the best healers in the world—Lori M., Tom, Christy, Alma, Peggy, Janet, and Michelle. They not only accept me for me, but celebrate and appreciate my authentic self. Our friendship spans decades and so many stories. A colleague even organized a meal drive when I was going through my divorce. I appreciate Hannah's friends' mothers like Holly, Sarah, Lisa, Andrea, and Becky for sharing their daughters and son to help a struggling little girl with social challenges get plenty of practice with friendships. The parents of Connor's friends have made sure he can build his own life and never feel as if he's in his sister's shadow. They, too, are warriors in my life, beefing up an area where it's hard for me to supply every need. Whether I'm teaching or the kids are with their dad, these moms text me pictures of Connor on field trips, participating in special school activities, and at Boy Scout events. Warriors fight for us and fill the gaps.

Don't be afraid to ask friends you work with or the parents of your child's friends to help with something. People often don't offer help because they don't know we need it. If we simply reach out with a specific request, they are often more than happy to help. Sometimes the most surprising warriors are people we barely know or people we know only in one context—maybe they are another tae kwon do parent and we've only sat at our kids' practices together. Maybe you see them hauling their child from the same school yours attends and dropping them off at the same art studio.

You might ask and someone will make excuses and avoid jumping in. That's okay. But some will surprise you by doing far more than you ever asked or imagined. You may find some good people and great friends.

THE CLOSEST WARRIORS

In the end, I have found that my warriors love my kids and me unconditionally—in happy times and hard times. They support us with the wisdom of a scholar and the gentleness of a nursemaid. All we have to do is allow them to give us their time, attention, and help, and receive it without apology. These women and men became my strength and fueled my courage to continue on. They fight for me, but they also give me a safe place to fall, providing a kind of safety net. And that net has helped me get rested and back on track for a better today and tomorrow.

And now, after years of reaching out for support, I am in a different place. I'm not as needy and don't have to rely on babysitters and childcare. We see fewer therapists and medical appointments are more spread out. Life is saner, and I think I'm stronger—strong enough, in fact, I often have enough to give to others. What a feeling to finally be able to give back and be a warrior for people who need me.

Others have witnessed my transformation with strength and grace and acknowledged their admiration. I have learned that, in general, individuals have great respect for women who have had things go wrong in their lives and have handled it like a warrior. Now, others are coming to me for empowering strategies.

You don't have to go it alone. Let someone know what you need (if you're just starting off on your journey, you could share the "10 Things You Can Do for a Parent Whose Child Just Received an Autism Diagnosis" list on page 200 to give them ideas). People are more willing to help than you might think. Find your warriors.

10 THINGS YOU CAN DO FOR A PARENT WHOSE CHILD JUST RECEIVED AN AUTISM DIAGNOSIS

- Don't judge. Trust me, she knows better than anyone else what to do, and she knows her child best. Only offer suggestions if she asks for them.
- Offer to help, and mean it. Whatever she needs, try to be there for her, and be there multiple times.
- Initially, don't send her research. She'll be logging a few million hours on the Internet without needing any extra articles.
- Never compare her child to your second cousin's neighbor's high school sweetheart's child with autism.
- Don't tell her he'll grow out of it. He'll make progress, but autism is a lifelong neurological disorder.
- Make them a meal. Having a meal waiting for us was a bright spot in our days when facing meltdowns, sleep-lessness, and mounds of paperwork for early interven-tion and school placements. Make the effort.
- If you know of anyone with a child with autism who might be a positive support for your friend, introduce them.
- Just listen. Don't share with your friend that your neu-rotypical child had sleeping/eating/behavioral issues, too. You have no idea how long your friend/family member might be dealing with these challenges. Just be there as a sounding board.
- Get both parents out. Find a way for them to enjoy a peaceful dinner or a movie once a month. It can help them as individuals and their marriage immensely.

Wisdom from the Round Table

Lori R.: Mrs. Jones dedicated six years of her career at Hickory Elementary as Cameron's one-on-one aide. *Words cannot capture* our deepest gratitude for what this amazing lady did for our son. Without a doubt, she was placed there by God.

Jen: Mr. Richard came along at just the right time. He was hired two weeks prior to sixth grade. I was nervous at first because we'd never had a male paraprofessional. That was exactly what Noah needed. Mr. Richard took Noah under his wing and was not only his paraprofessional, but he became Noah's friend and is like family. Mr. Richard took interest in what worked and didn't for Noah in many situations. He cared about Noah's education and to this day, eight years later, Noah and Mr. Richard have a fantastic friendship. When Noah sees him, his face lights up like it's Christmas morning. He was and is a true blessing to our family.

Lori V.: I was never fond of asking for help, but I had to learn to in order to survive. My friends have saved me on many occasions, and they have encouraged me to take time for me. Overall, though, one individual stands out and that was Byron's gymnastics coach. That man just naturally got it. His ability to help Byron feel welcome has been unparalleled! His gym was a safe haven for Byron and a fun place to be. This man was Byron's support, confidante, friend, and coach. To this day, Byron (now twenty-two) and he have a wonderful bond. In a world where Byron navigates without many friends, this man has been there. I will be eternally grateful to him.

Susan: Tyler has had amazing warriors as teachers over the years. We've been very fortunate to have such great teachers and therapists. I would also give credit to Meaningful Day Services. They have been so patient with our family as we go through troubling times. Our behavioral consultant, Patrick, has been outstanding. Without him, we may not be where we are today. He was instrumental in getting us to see outside our home and look into Tyler's future. As long as we've been together, he is really like part of the family. My friends and co-workers have also been with me throughout this journey. They have laughed with me, cried with me, carried me when I couldn't go any longer, and prayed for me. I could not have continued working had it not been for those ladies who have been around me all these years.

Karen: The good Lord always put the right person in our path that we needed.

Sarah: My husband and I had planned a trip out of town to celebrate our anniversary. My mom was going to keep the kids for the weekend, but the night before we left she came down with the flu. I scrambled around and was able to patch together a group of friends who would take turns watching the kids so we could still get away, but when I told Mitchell about it he almost lost it! He was upset that the plan had changed, and he was angry he wouldn't be with his siblings while we were away. I called my best friend and lamented to her. She told me to call all my friends back and let them know my kids would be with her for the entire weekend. Even though she had her hands full and plans of her own that weekend, she dropped everything to allow my husband and me a weekend away. She made the weekend fun and comfortable, accommodating all of my son's needs, so we could rest that he was well taken care of.

CHAPTER TWELVE

autism anecdotes

It takes a village to raise a child. It takes a child with autism to raise the consciousness of the village.

—Elaine Hall

September 2016

Today, my teaching partner and friend, Lori, and I are rolling out our version of Genius Hour *to our team of approximately sixty sixth graders.* Genius Hour *is a movement that allows students to explore their passions and encourages creativity in the classroom. It provides students with a choice in what they learn during a set period of time during school. There's also an undertone embedded within the movement to serve, help others, or impart knowledge. The project reminds me of Kevin Spacey's movie* Pay It Forward.

As students make their way back from related arts classes, we direct them into our team's science lab. Students scurry to find seats either in chairs at the lab tables or around the perimeter of the room, sitting on the lab stations' countertops. My daughter, Hannah, is one of those students. As she's progressed on the autism spectrum over the years, she's been mainstreamed into regular classrooms, having been re-diagnosed with Asperger's syndrome before it was removed from DSM-5.

Lori and I had not asked specifics from last year's teachers, so we begin by questioning our students. The last student we call on is one of the most vocal of our gifted/High Ability team. When he talks, everyone listens—they may not agree, but they listen. In fact, a week ago I'd pulled him into the hallway to compliment him for his incredible gift of saying things in the classroom that need to be said—things that I, as a teacher, probably shouldn't be saying. I appreciate his filtered comments and let him know his voice makes a difference.

Tall and thin, he has a pedantic presence complete with glasses. He stands, adjusts his glasses, and tells us his project last year included a study on obsessive-compulsive disorder (OCD). His research led him to a list of neurological disorders that could be associated with OCD (comorbidities). On that list he found autism.

With impeccable elocution, he begins:

"I moved here in fourth grade. Being in the high-ability cohort, everyone else had interacted with Hannah for years. I had not. It's no secret that the two of us didn't get along at all. The other kids shared with me that she had autism, but what is that? And does she really have it? Is it just gossip or maybe even an excuse to act the way she does? I went home and complained to my parents about our arguments, and I'm sure she did the same.

"You see, Hannah sees everything one way—it's black or white. There is no gray or anything in between. She is strong in her convictions and will defend them with earnest intensity. It's hard for her to understand that others can have a different point of view or opinion and that it's okay to disagree. Her headstrong personality only sees one way to get things done—her way. She's brutally honest to others, and it often seems as if she has no regard for their feelings. Other kids would let this go, but I simply could not."

This young man's insight into himself and Hannah astounds me. I listen as he shifts into another phase of understanding: awareness, which he articulates with understanding beyond his years. "I then read the symptoms in the book associated with autism. Hannah had so many of the listed symptoms. Hannah has challenges I can't even comprehend. I then became bothered and troubled. I felt sorry for her. I guess the words 'neurological' and 'disorder' hit me hard. Hannah has this malady and can't help it. It's how her brain is wired."

I hang on every word. Is this really happening? Why is a camera not rolling? "Hannah and I don't argue anymore, and I have her back—like everyone else." I can't believe how easily he progresses into a powerful phase: acceptance. He even uses the word! "I accept that she thinks and feels differently, but I also know it's important for her to fit in. I've learned how to talk to her, and I'm learning that what I once thought of as opinionated and bossy was her version of determined and driven. I would go so far as to call her my friend. That's what came out of my Genius Hour."

I sit—stunned.

What can I possibly say? He's just expressed my core belief—my mantra. I want all people to move from honest expressions of anger—or whatever emotion they're experiencing—to awareness and acceptance.

As Hannah's mom, I want to give that boy the biggest hug ever! But as Hannah's teacher, I know better. I decide to look at my daughter and gauge her reaction. She shifts slightly on the countertop and speaks up.

"No one has said anything that sweet before about my autism. What you just said really means a lot to me."

My teaching partner, Lori, walks over to the boy. She takes him by the hand to share and celebrate his epiphany with our administrators. I'll call his mother tomorrow to extend my appreciation.

I hope all the kids in the lab today can carry the message of awareness and acceptance into adulthood—into a world that needs people with insight and compassion toward others.

Because our children on the spectrum see the world through a different lens, as parents we can unlock our children's view by sharing stories so others may understand. And when we hear another parent share an experience similar to ours, it makes a scene or event that felt bizarre and outrageous suddenly seem more normal—and we feel less alone.

An autism parent has to be ready at all times with strategies to defuse situations and manage moods. Others think we should relax, but we know all hell could break loose at any moment over the smallest incident—and we are the only ones who can make everything okay. I used to jump every time the phone would ring. Sharing stories—autism anecdotes—can help the world understand our tension and vigilance— it's a way to spread awareness and advocacy!

The stories that follow may sound familiar. I encourage you to journal your own stories surrounding autism. You think you'll remember them, but you won't. Having a record of your journey will help you put the pieces together later and appreciate how much your child has emerged. I know it has helped me.

HOW TO PEEL A BANANA

Hannah has insisted on bringing the same lunch to school every day since kindergarten. Her usual restricted meal consists of a peanut butter and jelly sandwich, cinnamon applesauce, fruit snacks, a Reese's peanut butter cup, and a Capri Sun. No, it's not my idea of a healthy lunch, but when you have a child like Hannah, you're glad to get calories into her.

In the fall of 2016, Hannah's sixth grade year, I decided to slip a banana into her lunchbox. Hannah loves bananas, so I thought this would be an excellent idea.

While driving to school that morning, Hannah said, "Mom, I saw what you did! You thought I didn't see you, but I did. You put a banana into my lunchbox, and I am not going to eat it. You know I have to have the same thing packed every day!"

"I thought you'd tolerate the banana, since you like them so much."

"Mom, I am not going to be embarrassed around my friends because there's a banana in my lunchbox! You know that you've never taught me to peel a banana."

I drove in silence for a moment, realizing what I already suspected— that Hannah has never learned anything on her own by either watching others or trying to figure it out for herself.

Upon arriving in my classroom that morning, Hannah and I sat down and she learned how to peel a banana—adding another item she would tolerate in her lunchbox from then on.

HOW TO SAVE A LIFE

As I have mentioned in earlier chapters, aquatic therapy worked wonders for Hannah. She took aquatic therapy along with swim lessons throughout the year because the pressure soothed her body, and we were afraid, since she was a runner, that water was a safety hazard. By the time Hannah was in first grade, she was a top-notch swimmer. One evening, as we entered the pool area, we were told that there may be times that Hannah and her instructor would need to evacuate the pool due to mock lifesaving drills. Apparently, the lifeguards were being tested.

After I helped Hannah change into her swimsuit in the locker room, she headed to the diving well as usual. Hannah's instructor always allowed Hannah a few jumps off the low dive by herself while the instructor was changing. Connor and I found a seat in the bleachers, where I began making small talk with other parents.

Before I knew it, I heard several whistles blow. My eyes went directly to the diving well, where the lifeguards were quickly converging. I knew I would need to tell Hannah to get out of the water if her instructor was still in the locker room. However, as I looked out to the middle of the diving well, Hannah had a hand raised out of the water and her body was splashing water madly. Any other parent would be fearful that their child was in distress, but I knew exactly what was going on.

A lifeguard dove into the water with an orange lifesaving device in hand. He swam out to Hannah, placed her into a hold with his right arm from behind, and safely hauled her to the wall before two others lifted her out.

Hannah had heard and understood completely that the lifeguards would be doing mock drills that day—and she believed everyone was to participate. At this age, Hannah still had a tough time with receptive and expressive language, but her instructor and I were able to convince the staff that Hannah was a proficient swimmer and misunderstood the drill. This, unfortunately, did not excuse me from the lengthy accident report needed to document the incident.

THE MAN ON THE PLANE

Two years ago, after getting away to write, I boarded a flight from Ft. Myers to Charleston. As I sat down, I knew right away that the twenty-something sitting right beside me had autism. Yes, with all of our experiences, parents with children on the spectrum are blessed with an autism radar. I had the outside seat, and he immediately asked me to switch seats so there wouldn't be a chance that he would accidentally touch arms with people on both sides. Of course I agreed.

Without prompting, he said he was catching a connecting flight in Charleston to his parents' home in Dallas. "Living on my own didn't work out the way my family had hoped."

He fidgeted throughout the flight and couldn't relax. Then he misplaced his wallet. As he looked and shared his concern, I told him not to worry.

"You'll find it," I assured him. "I lose things all the time, and about the time I panic is when I find whatever was missing."

Sure enough, he found his wallet in one of his several pant pockets. Shortly after, he got into the overhead stowaway bin for a bottle of pills located in his carry-on. Earlier in our flight, he had scrunched a Starbucks cup and stuffed it into the pocket in the back of the seat in front of him. Now, he tried to straighten it out and used the remaining drink to swallow one of his pills. Throughout our one-hour flight, he went to the restroom five times. When paying for a bag of Chex Mix, he asked the exact size of the bag before spending his money.

As soon as the plane landed, he quickly called his mom, and they went over the directions for what to do next. He was so worried. After finishing his phone conversation, he explained that a wheelchair (even though he said he really didn't need one) would meet him when he deplaned and take him to his next gate because of his disability.

"Have a seat," I said as gently as possible. "I'll make sure the flight attendant takes very good care of you." After a pause, I said, "It's Asperger's, isn't it?"

"It's autism with an anxiety disorder."

On my way out, I told the flight attendant to take care of this young man. "He needs extra attention and patience to get to the wheelchair that will be waiting," I said.

As I exited the jet bridge and headed into the terminal's concourse, the tears flowed. The lump in my throat grew heavier and heavier as I passed the food court where I'd planned to eat dinner. I couldn't help but imagine my Hannah in a few years facing similar situations. Would she be as scared and anxious? Would she struggle to stay calm? *Would the person sitting next to her on the plane practice the same courtesy and compassion?*

DOESN'T HE KNOW THAT'S ANNOYING?

My ex-mother-in-law was always in Hannah's corner when it came to her autism. She and her husband would come to Indiana to support Hannah during the autism walks and even participate on their own in their home state of New York. They would send us pictures of their advocacy in local walks—in one, we saw the shirts they wore with Hannah's picture printed on the front. I would receive article after article in the mail she clipped related to autism.

Only once did she send a piece of mail I didn't appreciate. Not long after Hannah's diagnosis, my mother-in-law attended a colloquium focused on autism. One of the presentations concentrated on the five stages of grief parents experience after learning their child is on the spectrum—the stages paralleled grief associated with *death*. She sent me her notes. Although the paper was accurate, it was too soon for me to be hit with the information—I didn't want to know parenting Hannah would feel similar to grief over a death! The note upset me, but it wasn't my mother-in-law's fault. People have no way of determining how we'll emotionally process information.

Late one summer afternoon, the same in-laws wanted to take the kids to our subdivision's pool only four houses away. My husband wasn't home from work yet, so I thought this sounded like a great way to pass time. As we entered the pool area, I saw Blake in the pool. A tall, thin fourteen-year-old, Blake and his family lived across the street, and I knew Blake from when he attended our school. Blake's autistic behaviors included erratic flapping of his arms and a loud repetition of the same phrases over and over again (perseverative speech) to his grandmother, who was sitting under the canopy. This bothered no one else in the pool area, because everyone knew Blake and accepted his behaviors.

My ex-mother-in-law, however, didn't understand what was going on. "What is wrong with that young man? Doesn't he know he's annoying everyone?"

"No," I explained quietly, once more an advocate for people on the spectrum. "Blake doesn't know. He has autism, and autism doesn't manifest itself the same in any two people. It looks different for everyone."

She nodded, and I saw how open she was to learning more about autism. She grew to become a more informed autism advocate that day and has been more careful and compassionate with her words ever since.

I'VE SEEN A CUTER DOG

Last year, Hannah, Connor, and I decided that it was time to get a small dog. A friend of mine had posted photos on Facebook of their dog and explained how wonderful it was with her entire family. The dog was gorgeous! After researching the Cavapoo breed, I contacted my friend. We were able to set up a time for our family to visit with their beloved dog. In the meantime, we messaged back and forth about specific breeders, prices, and additional costs for having a dog. We had never owned one, so we gathered as much information as possible. And truth be told, I wanted a dog as much as the kids did. I couldn't wait for the visit!

The day came for us to see the dog. My friend's entire family was home and so proud to share stories. I had honestly never seen a cuter dog. We played with the dog for a while, and I could tell that Hannah and Connor were in awe. So I asked, "Well, Hannah, don't you think their dog is cute?"

"Yes," she said, "Rosie is cute. But my art teacher's dog is even cuter!"

Hannah is going to give her opinion no matter what.

We continue to work hard with her behavioral therapist to help Hannah tease out what is appropriate to say and what is not. Some people believe children who have autism don't possess empathy, but I disagree. I know Hannah is empathetic—I've seen her reach out to a friend in pain or stop an injustice. The challenge is to help her take an extra beat or two before she speaks to think about how her words will affect the person on the other end. In other words, she exhibits emotional or affective empathy, but still struggles with cognitive empathy. Although, more often than not, when Hannah is told that she has hurt another's feelings, there is deep remorse and regret. She never fails to care when she knows, but all too often she doesn't know when she needs to care.

WANT TO MAKE YOUR MOTHER HAPPY?

Until about five years ago, I believed that people with autism were more capable of understanding others' emotions than many of us gave them credit for. I held firm to this belief until I had a conversation with a student of mine with Asperger's syndrome.

Derek was having a horrible time in the evenings trying to focus on homework. His mother claimed that ten grade-level computation problems in math could take hours. Assuming this was true, we'd have to adjust his workload. His case conference committee determined that in order to be excused from the nightly assignments, Derek would need to do two of the problems during the school day to prove mastery to me.

One day not long after his committee's meeting, I prompted Derek at least three times to complete the problems during seatwork. Instead, he kept folding little squares of paper in half. After class was released, I spoke with Derek in the hallway. I tried to explain how his lack of attention meant he would have homework in the evening. He stared at the floor, listening but unable to make eye contact.

"This isn't going to make your mother happy, Derek. If you can find the time in another teacher's class today to complete the problems, I'll look at them and excuse you from the evening's homework."

He looked up, but only stared and said nothing. I wanted to make sure he heard my offer. "Now, Derek, think of how much better that would make your mother feel. That would make your mother happy. If you do the problems in one of your classes today, the two of you wouldn't need to focus on math homework tonight. Doesn't it make you feel good when your mother is happy?"

Nothing. I got nothing from him but a blank, emotionless gaze. As smart as Derek was, he couldn't connect with what I was saying. Derek was a kind, sweet-hearted boy toward others in the classroom and toward me. He meant no malice toward his mother by his apparent disinterest. To me, it was anecdotal evidence of **mind-blindness**. In other words, "If I can't/don't feel it or perceive it, then they can't/don't feel it or perceive it."

TIME TO CHANGE CLOTHES

The summer after Hannah's kindergarten year, she attended our zoo's week-long summer day camp. These camps were valuable for two reasons. First, they kept Hannah on a strict schedule, which is vital to create stability for kids on the spectrum. Second—and most important over the long run—they allowed her to embrace her affinity with animals in a social setting with other children.

Connor and I walked into the zoo's education center, and as I signed Hannah out at the front desk, the woman told me that the director asked to speak privately with me. I couldn't imagine what he was about to say.

Hannah, he said, had committed an infraction.

Since it was an extremely hot day, the staff had taken the campers to the zoo's splash park. I knew this was a possible activity, so I'd made sure to have Hannah wear her suit under her regular clothes to simplify the process of changing. We had methodically reviewed the steps needed to slip out of the suit's arm straps in order to use the restroom. However, once again, I hadn't done enough.

When the splash pad activities were completed, the camp counselor had told the kids, "Okay, now it's time to change." Hannah took this to mean it was time to change at that very second. Without a thought, she slipped her bathing suit off and stood in front of campers, counselors, and a few zoo visitors.

The director's stern face told me I should be appalled, but I was thinking, "I know, I know this is wrong. I don't really care people saw her naked because that's not the biggest issue." I said all the right things, though, and promised to review the situation with her. Life has always been like this with Hannah. Maybe I'm numb to the embarrassment or lack of social pragmatics, but Hannah's behavior didn't faze me. If someone says it's time to get changed, *of course* Hannah is going to undress as soon as she's able to process the words.

I did as I promised the director—I reviewed with Hannah that we never, ever undress in public or in front of others. I also reminded her to continue to watch others and draw cues from them—what we infer and what is meant could be two different things. I think she understood. She's been to the zoo camp every year since then during some of the hottest days of summer, and I've never again had to face the director to hear about an incident of public indecency.

TIME FOR OUR FAMILY TO ESCAPE

A few years ago, the three of us went to a friend's family's Labor Day cookout. She and her husband have three children, one of whom is Connor's age. It was extremely warm outside, so the kids were playing with water guns. Hannah had reached the age and independence level that she was fine alone with other children.

A girl about four years younger than Hannah was squirting her, but would not allow Hannah to do the same. Hannah insisted this was not okay, but I explained, "She's younger, so just don't spray her, Hannah."

As the day went on, the kids dried off and went upstairs to play in the family's loft, which overlooked their family room. We were able to glance up at the kids and hear if something happened. Out of nowhere we heard the little girl's scream. All I heard was "Hannah!" I raced upstairs. The little girl was holding her arm, and Hannah was apologizing over and over and over. I still remember her look of distress and remorse. No one saw what happened except the two of them. Hannah said the little girl wanted something Hannah had, so the little girl pushed her. Hannah then hit the little girl on the arm. The way the little girl was crying it must have been hard.

The parents had been outside and appeared in no time. The parents looked at me and said that my daughter had been taunting their daughter at the party for some time now, and because of this, they were leaving. They then told me I needed to keep my daughter on a shorter leash.

I was flabbergasted someone would talk this way. I also knew that Hannah had not been aggravating their daughter. I apologized up and down anyway and told them that we would be the ones to leave.

My friend asked me to please stay. She didn't know what the couple had said to me. I just apologized to her, put the kids in the car, and escaped.

Hannah shouldn't have hit the girl in retaliation, so we were not entirely in the right, but this was not our fault and we weren't the only people who should have apologized. And yet, sometimes we must end a situation swiftly and do what makes us feel secure. At that moment I knew I needed out of that scene, so I got us out!

YOU MUST CHECK IN BEFORE ENTERING

Hannah used to attend the school where I teach, so she walked into and out of school with me every day. There's a sign on the second set of inside doors to our school that reads, You Must Check in at The Front Office Desk Before Entering the Building. The first day of school, Hannah entered and stopped after the first set of doors, adamant that we weren't allowed past the second set of doors without checking in with the office first.

She began yelling, "Stop, Mom! You can't just walk through there." I tried to explain that the sign was for students or adults who don't teach in the building, but she would have none of my explanation. To Hannah, rules are to be strictly enforced, not interpreted.

So we went into the office, and I asked the secretaries to tell Hannah assertively and without a doubt that it was okay for the both of us to walk through the doors every morning without checking in at the main office. I know the secretaries didn't understand the need to intensely express their permission, and it used to bother me that people might think I'm overly vigilant, but I've come to terms with it. I needed to—it's how I survive with my daughter who processes the world differently.

It worked. Hannah and I continued to successfully pass through the second set of doors all 360 days of her career at my school without checking in at the main office.

HIS NAME IS COLIN

It was fall of 2017 and Hannah was now in the seventh grade. I had arrived at cross country practice to pick her up, and Hannah immediately started complaining that Connor was sitting in the front seat. She and Connor quarrelled for a while before she asked what was for dinner. When I responded with "Chili," that wasn't good enough. After walking into our home, Hannah refused to get her all her things—backpack, laptop case, violin case, lunchbox—out of the car. That became my job.

Throughout the evening, her behavior didn't improve one bit. Homework, piano practice, shower time, and our nightly devotional were all a struggle. I had listened to enough. She had set the tone of our entire evening, and I wasn't going to allow her to behave like this one more time.

This is exactly when the epic "Mommy fail" happened. I had lost my patience. Nothing I could do for her was good enough, nor were my prompts being acknowledged. She did not have the right to speak to me in such a condescending tone! Who was this child? I self-diagnosed this as "tween" behavior versus autism. Right then and there, I looked at her and said, "Since I can't seem to do anything right for you, I believe it's time for you to take care of yourself!" And then I knew I had to follow through.

I instructed her on how to set her alarm clock to awaken for school the next day all by herself. I then reminded her of the three lists posted in the house that sequenced her morning routine: on the bathroom cabinet door, on the kitchen breakfast table, and on the laundry room door. I reminded her that her bus arrives at 6:42 sharp, and she would need to catch it because I wasn't going to take her to school. As soon as my head hit the pillow that evening, I knew I had made a mistake. What was I thinking?

Her alarm sounded at 5:45. My bedroom is in the same hallway as hers, so I knew I could listen to her every move. She nonchalantly came into my room and whispered, "I'm up, Mom, and I'm going to get ready." Next, I heard her in the bathroom brushing her teeth and opening and closing the bathroom drawers. I then listened to her walk downstairs to her list. The refrigerator was opened along with the pantry door. *Could she really be doing this herself?*

After listening to her eat breakfast, I heard her scurry to get all of her bags and cases sorted. The garage door went up, and I heard a "Bye, Mom," to which I replied that I loved her very much and to have a good day. Why was I smiling? Did Hannah really complete her morning routine without my help? Then I remembered the jacket.

Hannah would be so cold at the bus stop without her jacket! Would she remember that I always keep an extra in her backpack? I flew down the hallway to Connor's room, peeked through the blinds, and I saw Hannah at the bus stop. She put down her backpack and other belongings, pulled out her jacket and put it on, and then packed up again! She hopped on the bus, and my phone dinged with her text: "I'm sorry, Mom. It won't happen again." A mother's "epic fail" had turned into her daughter's success! But that's not all.

As I picked Hannah up after cross country practice that day, she said, "Mom, his name is Colin." I had no idea what she was talking about. I asked her, and she said that Colin was the name of the boy who stands at the bus stop with her every morning.

She finally remembered. I had been asking her for the past two weeks to find out the name of the boy at the bus stop. She didn't consider his name important to her, so she hadn't asked. She knew it was important to me, and she finally asked. A mistake by me became a shining success for Hannah, and it spoke volumes about the progress she was making toward independence.

THE WORLD THROUGH A DIFFERENT LENS

I could fill three more chapters with anecdotes unique to the autism experience, but I'll leave you with one of my favorites—the time Hannah told me that no one else's peanut butter and jelly sandwich tastes like mine. I've seen this same incident occur on the television show *Parenthood,* when Max's father offered to make him a sandwich for his school lunch. Max denied his father the favor, arguing that it wouldn't be the same as Mom's.

I hope that you, too, are able to derive some delight in our children's peculiarities, even as they unfold in the midst of struggles and tears. These stories remind us how our children interpret the world—and how lucky are we, as their parents, to be privy to their lens.

TIPS FOR SUPPORTING SOCIAL INTERACTIONS[25]

- Extend a feeling of welcome and model for other participants that the child with autism is a valued part of the group.
- Get to know the child with autism and meet him where he currently is in terms of social skills and interests.
- Be aware that free play or other unstructured times are the most difficult for people with autism. Think about how to impose some structure on these activities.
- People with autism often have a difficult time maintaining eye contact. Insisting on eye contact can cause additional stress.
- Children with autism, especially those who are more verbal, can be the target of teasing and bullying. They often do not pick up on nonverbal cues such as tone of voice or the hidden intention of a request or comment. They often go along with the teasing or bullying because they do not identify that it has a negative

intent. Their desire to make friends coupled with their difficulty doing so means they often encounter peers with negative intentions. Be on the lookout for this and respond quickly if teasing or bullying becomes an issue.

❖ Many people with autism are very logical and will always play according to the rules. If the rule is that basketballs are not allowed outside at a particular time, a participant may become agitated if they come out for a special activity. Similarly, he may not understand special circumstances in game play such as penalty shots, and his insistence on following the rules he has learned could become problematic.

❖ Identify peers who model strong social skills and pair the child with autism with them. Provide peers with strategies for eliciting communication, but be careful not to turn the peer into a teacher. Strive to keep peer interactions as natural as possible.

❖ During group activities, define his role and responsibilities within the group. Assign a role or help him mediate with peers as to what he should do. Rotate roles to build flexibility and broaden skills.

❖ If you leave it up to the group to pick partners, children with autism are sometimes chosen last, causing unnecessary humiliation. Develop a method that follows its own random pattern—pulling names from a bucket of popsicle sticks or pairing using birthdays works well.

✺ Wisdom from the Round Table ✺

Lori R.: I am going to preface my story by saying that our family had been watching the television show *The Biggest Loser*, and Cameron would express his disgust as the contestants would show their upper body at the weigh-ins. At a family reunion a few years ago, we were walking toward the shelter. Cam was several yards ahead of us and had to pass by a relative he had never met who was extremely large. I could see the wheels turning in Cam's head as he walked past the man and was looking directly at his body. I held my breath as Cam walked past him and sighed relief when Cam didn't say anything about this man being rather large. Before I could get to Cam, he turned around, went up to the man and asked, "So, how much do you eat anyway?"

I wanted to crawl in a hole, to say the least, but secretly celebrating that Cam had made the connection with overeating and obesity. The man replied, "Well, obviously I eat too much!" Cam replied back, "That's right!" Cam then walked away.

Jen: When Noah was younger, the summer before fourth grade, I made a summer schedule for him in order for the days to go more smoothly. I would type the numbered activities out on paper. I would fill in the numbers according to how the day would flow, but I would always put "surprise" in at least one or two of the blanks in case something came up that needed to be done. One day Noah filled in one of the blanks with IU (Indiana University) basketball. It was on a Saturday in June, and we knew that couldn't happen. But we loaded up the car, drove to Bloomington, and went to IU to show Noah the doors were locked. They were actually open! They were having basketball camp, so we went in and watched a little basketball, left, and checked that off the sheet.

Lori V.: When Byron was about four years old (pre-diagnosis), he was part of the youth Christmas play at church. He was one of the three wise men standing right in front. During the part where everyone was talking about what gift they had brought for baby Jesus, one of the angels recited her line, "I brought him a pillow to rest his weary head."

Byron piped up and said, "Aww, that's nice!" The congregation gave a small chuckle. The next child to speak said her line, and

Byron again spoke out and said, "That's so sweet!" The congregation couldn't hold back their laughter. Byron didn't understand
that they were laughing at his adorable commentary and immediately moved a step toward the congregation, his face totally in
meltdown preparation mode. He shook his fist and yelled at the
congregation, "Do you want a piece of me?" I was in the back with
my other son and couldn't get out to him; however, I could see the
shock and horror on his face. That was his first and last production.

Susan: We took Tyler to one of his neurology appointments when
he was almost ten. Our daughter, Allie, was with us. The doctor suggested that Tyler be put into an inpatient facility for a few
days due to his aggressive behavior. He was throwing such a fit,
and I felt so sorry for Allie. After the appointment, we went home
to pack a bag for Tyler. I will never forget the feeling of packing
his bag and wondering what was going to happen. Who would
know what he wants? He had so little communication. Who would
change his diaper? How will they make sure he gets his milk? All
these things were going through my mind while I was packing. The
tears just kept flowing. We then took Tyler back to the hospital for
the inpatient. We sat at a small cubicle as the social worker tried
to get Tyler into their facility. As she spoke with the insurance company, Tyler continued screaming, hitting, and biting. The insurance
denied payment for inpatient. The social worker tried and tried to
explain the situation. The insurance kept telling her that this is the
nature of autism spectrum disorder, which is not covered by insurance. She even stated, "I am sitting here watching him bite, hit,
and scream." The insurance wouldn't pay, so we went back home
with our son. The three of us were quiet in the house all night long
while we listened to Tyler's screaming.

Karen: When Eric was about three, he was into everything like
most three-year-olds. Once he pulled open the door of a hot oven,
and while I was yelling, "No!" he reached in and burned his hand.
I got his hand into cold water right away, but he still had blisters,
tears, and lots of pain. We talked about hot ovens, and he seemed

to understand. A while later, I had the oven on again. Same exact thing—he did it again. I couldn't believe it, but I realized if searing pain wouldn't stop his impulsivity, really nothing could. For years after, I didn't use the oven even with a lock because Eric could figure out how to bypass most safety devices.

Sarah: Although Mitchell doesn't like to write, his pragmatism was made evident in a poem he constructed about the sun at age ten. He used the paradoxical view that eventually the sun is going to kill us, but without it, the lack of heat would kill us anyway.

CHAPTER THIRTEEN

acceptance and fostering independence

We must be willing to get rid of the life we planned so as to have the life that's waiting for us.

—Joseph Campbell

November 2015

I'm teaching my sixth grade students how to systematically solve for a variable in a math equation, and I get a strange feeling I need to check on Hannah. What time is it? Where would she be?

Lunch. I have only walked through her lunch period once before, at the beginning of the year. I continue teaching, but something continues to bother me. Mother's intuition?

I assign a set of ten problems, have an aide watch my students, and rush to the cafeteria. I arrive and scan the tables. Most are full of kids laughing and leaning and swapping sandwiches. One table close to the kitchen entry catches my attention because it's so bare. There she is. My daughter, at a lunch table all by herself—sobbing. She hasn't touched her lunch.

I sit down.

"Mom," she says. "You see all of these kids? They all come into the cafeteria with at least one person in mind they want to sit with. Me? I have no one. They all talk so quickly, Mom, I can't understand their words. And their jokes, I really don't understand why they think they're funny."

"We will get this fixed," I say, frantically scanning the lunchroom for a table of considerate girls willing to share their table. A little girl gestures to me that Hannah is more than welcome to sit at their table. By now I can tell the lunch monitors are aware of the situation. Their eyes are on us. I tell Hannah that the girls want her to sit with them. She glances over and they smile. She picks up her tray and walks over. Crisis averted.

She only wants to belong. A child with high-functioning autism knows she's different and doesn't fit in. The anxiety can be debilitating. I know we'll face more crises.

But I'm relieved for the moment. And it occurs to me as I walk back to my classroom that my daughter has gained a skill we've worked on for years: she's learned to communicate her emotions.

I smile at that thought, then realize I need to make a mental list of what needs to be done to avoid this happening again:

. . . email the lunch supervisors asking them to intervene the next time Hannah is alone,

. . . talk with her teachers to see if they are willing to pair Hannah with someone for lunch,

. . . phone the autism consultant to create a personalized story that emphasizes how to find a seat with others,

. . . talk with the school counselor and ask her to discuss this problem with Hannah during "Friendship Group,"

. . . text her behavioral management specialist to discuss this with Hannah tonight.

I'll also text Hannah's dad, my ex-husband, to explain the situation. Has this happened before? Oh my, I pray not.

Now I need to walk into my classroom and pretend as if nothing has happened. I open the door.

"Okay, anyone need help?"

Hannah still faces significant challenges, such as social pragmatics; however, her gains over the last ten years have been extraordinary. She is now in a seventh grade High Ability Program and prospering! Educators refer to her diagnosis as being twice-exceptional (2e). This is an interplay between giftedness and autism. Individuals with Asperger's syndrome typically demonstrate these traits: average to above-average intelligence, social and communication deficits, obsessive and narrowly defined interests, concrete and literal thinking, inflexibility, problem-solving and organizational problems, difficulty in discerning relevant from irrelevant stimuli, and behavioral issues that are often related to lack of understanding.

FIVE VALUABLE LESSONS THAT FOSTER INDEPENDENCE FOR CHILDREN ON THE SPECTRUM

- Focus on life skills. What does every individual need to be able to do to function on their own? Start small and slowly increase complexity. It's never too early to start self-care skills. Don't allow learned helplessness. It takes time, but the benefits are worth your patience.
- Include chores around the home into the daily and weekly schedule. What can your child do to help around the house to increase self-worth, pride, and lend a helping hand?
- Provide your child with visual supports and tools to counteract those probable poor executive functioning skills. This takes time in the beginning, but once complete, motor planning and time management challenges are decreased. Lists and schedules pay off enormously.
- Make a list of skills outside of the home that our typical children have picked up just by watching us, and teach them to your child on the spectrum. Ideas include

knowing how to scan groceries, finding the appropriate shirt size in a clothing store, ordering from a menu, and more.

❖ Teach your child to stay safe in as many situations as you can imagine. Can they cross a street? Do they know to stay away from fire and water? Do they know not to talk (if verbal) to strangers or go with them?

GIRLS ON THE SPECTRUM

Aside from Temple Grandin, not much has been reported about girls on the spectrum. Most literature is based on the "blue side" of autism, because boys far outnumber girls diagnosed with autism spectrum disorders, with the ratio estimated at 4:1. However, identifying girls on the spectrum is critical. Life with autism is different for girls than it is for boys. In general, girls are expected to be social butterflies, to interact on a more personal level than boys, and understand social cues and facial expressions better than boys. I see evidence of this generalization every day in my classroom.

Not so for girls with autism.

At a very young age, I discovered that Hannah was oblivious to facial expressions. At the time, Hannah really enjoyed jigsaw puzzles. The special education teacher at our school allowed me to borrow a puzzle with several different facial expressions. After Hannah memorized the facial expressions' meanings, we then reviewed situations in which others would use those specific facial expressions. Creating concrete examples for Hannah brought more meaning and understanding to her world.

Girls on the spectrum may seem to prefer to spend their time alone, with animals, or with books, but this may not be true. In Hannah's case, she was simply confused by how to socially "fit in." She found boys less complicated because their play (LEGOs, Minecraft, and coding) was less social, more functional, and, therefore, more interesting to her. Given this, it's easy to see why her longtime best buddy is a boy. Hannah still takes on the role of "boss" to younger girls, needier children, and students new to her class. Before this past school year,

Hannah would gravitate toward the few individuals in each of her classes who also seemed not to fit in. For some reason, befriending these individuals allowed her to feel normal. And I needed to be okay with this. I will also add, as a sidenote, that a computer is not a replacement for a friend.

Hannah, like many girls with autism, is not as emotionally mature as others her age. In some areas she seems a few years behind. At the age of twelve, she is just now caring about the look of her hair, the brand of her clothes, makeup, and the latest fads while her peers have talked about these things for years. At times I wondered if she even got that others did things differently. I continue to explain to her that appearance does matter to some people. I'm not saying that apathy toward hairstyle, clothing brands, and fads is wrong—it's just different. Make sure you also help your child to understand that while they may not care about how they look, others may not want to interact with them because of this.

During the summer of 2015, I met Jennifer O'Toole at the Autism Society of America's national conference. Jennifer, founder of *Asperkids.com* and author of several *New York Times* bestsellers, including *Asperkids*, *The Asperkid's Secret Book of Social Rules*, and *Sisterhood on the Spectrum*, is giving parents with girls on the spectrum valuable and tangible resources. In *Sisterhood of the Spectrum: An Asperger Chick's Guide to Life*, she explains to fellow Aspies, "We often mistake our most immeasurable gifts for shameful flaws. You are lovable. Right now. Without changing a thing."[26] I see that and believe it—now I just need to be sure Hannah knows it. Every day, I want her to know how lovable she is right now, just as she is.

ALLOWING MY DAUGHTER TO BE HANNAH

I have shifted my mindset when it comes to Hannah. Until as recently as last year, I really thought I could "fix" Hannah 100 percent—as if she were broken or damaged! After over ten years of trying to make her more "normal" and fit the mold of what I thought I wanted in my beautiful daughter, I peacefully and providentially realized that my daughter was hardwired to be exactly who she is every day. I thought I'd "fix"

Hannah, but she taught me acceptance. Emerging from autism does not mean she's healed from autism or rescued from autism or "fixed." That was not my intent with the word "emerging." What I discovered is all the hard work has freed her from assumptions medical professionals had made. They assumed she would be unable to integrate with the world, but she has. I've come to realize she has emerged from limitations and constraints, but she has autism and always will, and that's part of what makes her beautiful. It makes your child beautiful too! Hannah needs my love, not someone she feels as if she can't please.

I have a tough, spitfire human being on my hands. I have a strong and powerful daughter to raise. She didn't need fixing—I did! I needed to fix my perception of my daughter and autism. The girl right in front of me revels in watching *Jeopardy*, dispensing obscure bits of animal trivia, leaving her shoes untied, and incessantly arguing the "why" of math problems until I'm out of answers. This is the girl I have—this is the girl I want! What we may find most endearing about our children on the spectrum could actually be attributed to their autism, and that is certainly the case with myself and Hannah.

I've learned to see her for what she is. A slight spin on some of the traits I used to find frustrating—attached, blunt, opinionated, strong and bossy—helped me see Hannah as loyal, honest, passionate, driven, and ambitious. I had been fighting too much with her inner being—the person she was truly meant to be. I was stretching her, which is not all bad, but I started to see that if I stretched a little too far at age twelve, her true spirit would break. I never, ever want to convey the feeling of shame onto my daughter. How freeing for us both when I saw this and shifted how I interacted with her. Hannah says, "Mom, I'm like a Skittle in a Mason jar full of M&M's."

Author Paul Collins wrote, "Autists are the ultimate square pegs, and the problem with pounding a square peg into a round hole is not that the hammering is hard work. It's that you're destroying the peg."[27] I never want to destroy or diminish Hannah's self-confidence. Temple Grandin has said we should be teaching people with autism to adapt to the social world around them while still retaining the essence of who they are, including their autism. Hannah and I are learning to accept, embrace, and even, as much as possible, celebrate her autism. Find ways in which you can do this with your child. I am positive that is one of the reasons why Hannah does allow her story to be told.

Be the Skittle in a Mason jar full of M&M's, Hannah. Without changing a thing.

Hannah is exactly who she was meant to be. I want to equip Hannah with a positive attitude and self-esteem. She doesn't need to mask her identity or feel as if she needs to blend in. I don't want depression or a poor self-image to rob her of her gifts. I celebrate her spirit and encourage her passions—though they differ wildly from my own. I want her to have a fulfilling life. Encouraging Hannah's passions has provided a life raft for the both of us. Her anxiety levels decrease during these activities, which directly affects her behavior. Dr. Barry Prizant, author of *Uniquely Human*, said, "Though they come with challenges, enthusiasms often represent the greatest potential for people with autism. What begins as a strong interest or passion can become a way to connect with others with similar interests, a lifelong hobby, or, in many cases, a career." Continue to encourage your child's passions—even if you don't share the enthusiasm. I highly recommend Dr. Prizant's book.

Less than a year ago, Hannah attended a veterinarian camp at our local zoo. Before my realization, I never would have allowed her to miss school for this. Now I want to nurture her interests, so I sent her to the camp. I received texts all day—photos of her examining X-rays, observing a surgery, and studying anatomy. Those were the first texts I had ever received from my daughter. She only took the phone to take pictures. And now, when she thinks of it or when I prompt her, she texts friends and there's often a short exchange. It's surprising to see how light-hearted and fun her texts appear in comparison to her everyday verbal communication. Hannah is allowing her passion to become her purpose, and it's made a marked difference in her level of socialization and our view of the future.

I'll never forget the taxi cab driver I met over a year ago while on a short working vacation. In the middle of me explaining my need for respite, Kevin stopped at a light, turned around, smiled, and gently said, "It gets better as they age. I have a son with autism at home that's twenty-eight. He was diagnosed at four years of age just after his mother passed away. Here's what I tell everyone about acceptance. One morning I woke up and found that our circumstances were fine—no more trying to change my son. It takes a while, though."

FINDING NEW WAYS TO CORRECT BEHAVIORS

Along with this epiphany has come a new way of directing and correcting some of Hannah's behaviors—social gaffes that are hindering where she wants to be in life. I do accept Hannah for who she is, but when she makes others think they are less—even if she is oblivious to the impact of her words and actions—I want to find ways she can monitor and shift what she's doing and saying. I know she can be a voice of kindness and support for others, so I have been working with her on building awareness. I have found that it's absolutely necessary to not only correct a behavior but also to explain why the behavior is not acceptable. This helps Hannah understand, adopt, and utilize the new rule. I heard John Elder Robison, author of *Be Different*, speak in the summer of 2017 about his family keeping up the fight, trying to train him in manners even if they made no sense to him. He said, "I benefited from social compliance. Asperger's syndrome causes me to be more logical and straightforward. Manners are neither." Being proactive is also beneficial. Explaining social "rules" to Hannah before she is expected to use them empowers her with direction. Rules make social situations more clear. It's also been important to explain which topics are conversations best left as private exchanges with appropriate individuals—public taboo. Make sure you make a point to take the time to do this with your child. If not, their social miscues will continue to cause them trouble.

Hannah has always known she has autism; we've never kept it a secret from her or anyone else. Yet we don't broadcast it to gain pity or special consideration. Hannah is now mature enough to understand that her autism produces certain behaviors like interrupting, turn-taking challenges, correcting, and perseverating on a topic—behaviors that can annoy or insult others. In our family's daily routine, I've even had to go as far as assigning Connor to family prayer and Hannah to riding shotgun on even days, and vice versa on odd days. This has worked, so

I assume her need to follow a "rule" trumps her challenge of turn-taking. Try something like this if you are having similar struggles.

We value courtesy and believe it is rude to correct an authority figure or elder, and yet Hannah does this—especially when correcting her grandparents' grammar. Antagonizing is another trait we continue to work on. Hannah becomes upset if people don't say "thank you," "you're welcome," and "bless you." She points out the mistakes, errors, and oversights of others like going over the speed limit, not washing hands after using the restroom, forgetting the blessing before dinner, and using foul language. She is a rule keeper. Hannah also corrects others when they answer "uh, huh" rather than "yes." In her mind, there is only a "yes" or a "no." In *Be Different*, Robison said, "I learned to accept the way other people do things even when I'm sure that they are wrong." With help and structure, I know Hannah will also make it to this point.

Hannah has made many social blunders by failing to filter her thoughts before verbalizing them. Her "filter" was allowing too much information through, which resulted in embarrassment—on my part, not hers.

It all started at age six. Our family had just finished eating at a local chain restaurant. While leaving the restaurant, Hannah paused at a couple's table. The man had a full beard and a mustache. She said, "I don't like your face." Another time, she walked up to a gentleman in a local superstore and asked him if he had seen the movie *Toy Story 2*. When he replied yes, I knew we were in trouble. She proceeded to tell him that he looked just like the chicken man—the antagonist of the movie who was a bit chubby and had a receding hairline.

Two years ago, while touring the U-505 submarine exhibit at the Museum of Science and Industry in Chicago, the docent asked our group of about fifteen if there were any questions before beginning the tour. Hannah raised her hand and asked the docent his or her gender. The docent nicely told Hannah to look at her nametag. Hannah said the docent's name aloud and then said, "Girl." I pulled Hannah aside to explain why this was rude, and said she needed to apologize. Hannah had no idea her actions were socially inappropriate. "Mom," she said, "if she doesn't want people to ask the question, then maybe she should try a little harder to look like a girl." Once again, my daughter approaches everything with a matter-of-factness that is inappropriate. I've learned that autism is a little like playing chess with Connor. I always need to think two to three steps ahead.

Hannah's counselor and I have worked on educating Hannah about how her comments affect how others feel. One of the best tactics I used when she was younger was one I got from our school system's autism consultant: Hannah's rule was that she could not talk to strangers, even if one of her parents was present, unless she asked us first.

SOCIAL SKILLS

Hannah struggles daily with our society's unwritten basic level of social interaction. In education, this is referred to as the **"hidden" curriculum**. She's been known to let a door shut behind her without holding it open for the next person. She used to also change the television channel while another member of the family was watching their favorite show and simply didn't understand why this was wrong. People expect cultural rules to be followed. Most children naturally pick up on them by watching others. Not Hannah.

My solution: When Hannah unwittingly commits a social faux pas, I pull her aside and explain that her autism doesn't allow her to understand why this social nuance is not acceptable, but others would see her behavior as embarrassing. I explain that she doesn't want others to feel uncomfortable or embarrassed by anything she says or does, so she and I have discussed how "embarrassing" feels and looks because she didn't typically experience this emotion. After all, how could she feel embarrassed by a behavior if she doesn't know it's unacceptable? Now that Hannah is twelve years old, she does know how embarrassing feels but doesn't always connect that what she's saying or doing is embarrassing. I did apparently manage to embarrass her a few times as her math and science teacher in sixth grade and heard about it. Actually, we all heard about it. I've found that helpful social hints are best received if given by Hannah's friends instead of an adult.

When Hannah attended the school where I teach, I witnessed her lack of social reciprocity when others greeted her in the hallway. I asked her about it and found out that Hannah was indeed saying "Hello," but not loud enough for anyone else to hear. She's had a similar issue with smiling: Her smile is sometimes perceived as a smirk. Then I learned the medical explanation for this. Scientists studying the brain have found that the brains of individuals with autism have weak **mirror neurons**. Mirror neurons are brain cells whose specific function is to "act out" what we see in other people. So if other people smile, typical functioning people will naturally smile back, whereas individuals with autism might smile only slightly. When others say "hello," some individuals with autism have replies that are barely audible. I'm trying to help Hannah understand this, so she can raise her self-awareness over time and adjust. Does she now grin at people when they smile at her? Does she consistently respond with a confident, pleasant "hello" when someone greets her? No. But I've heard her raise her volume a notch, and I've witnessed a subtle, Mona Lisa grin in response to a teacher's friendly wave. She's internalized these conversations and is making progress, and I'm proud of her for trying.

Another behavior has been known to agitate others. Hannah's ears are very sensitive to the sounds of people eating and drinking. Make too much noise, and Hannah is sure to let you know. And then, she'll monitor closely in fear of hearing the distressing sound again!

"Theory of mind" is the term coined for the ability to interpret one's own and others' mental and emotional states—understanding that each person has unique motives and perspectives. Hannah, like most individuals with autism, struggles to see that others have different perspectives. This is also known as mind-blindness. Be sure to check out Simon Baron-Cohen's "Sally-Anne test" for an activity that models this social cognitive challenge. Jennifer O'Toole calls Aspies "illiterate telepaths."[28] My confidence and compassion in discussing these behaviors with Hannah comes from a deep understanding of how my daughter operates. Hannah does truly have a need to fit in, have friends, and be accepted, so she agrees with the need to invest in trying to understand others' opinions.

Hannah is also a concrete, literal thinker. Early one morning, years ago, Hannah woke me up. Anxious and agitated, she held one of the *Diary of a Wimpy Kid* books in her hands and jumped into my bed.

"Mom, I am so sorry to wake you, but I have been up most of the night and still can't find it. Please help me find it, Mom."

I looked down at the book and saw the words "go back to square one." Hannah had stayed up most of the night and was up before the sun rose looking for a square with a one in or beside it, or a chapter named "Square One." My daughter is the most literal person I know. It's a common thread in children with autism that parents must be prepared for when speaking and giving directions.

Thankfully, she's learned in the years since then that idioms, clichés, sarcasm, metaphors, and other forms of figurative or nonliteral language exist, but even at age twelve she struggles to spot them and grasp their meanings. I found a kids' book on idioms to help her better understand language. We talked through each one and discussed what it meant, like "smart as a whip" and "knock your socks off." Her favorites were "It's raining cats and dogs" and "Has the cat got your tongue?" Leave it to cats to capture her attention. She memorized their implied meanings versus their literal meanings. I've found this to be an effective strategy, and one I'd recommend to parents.

It takes a lot of reminders, but every day Hannah is showing me that she can overcome, compensate for, and self-manage many of autism's most challenging characteristics. The more Hannah understands her autism, the better equipped she'll be with skills to enjoy a productive, independent adulthood. This has been particularly helpful to Hannah when trying to understand her own idiosyncrasies. For example, thoughts, words, and phrases still continue to get stuck in her mind on a loop, and they play over and over. She now understands that it's not possible for her to always sit in the same exact seat when playing violin in the orchestra. Understanding her autism allows her to take control of these type of episodes. Hannah says that she has to trick her brain to do something that everyone else sees as normal.

SOCIALIZATION

I'm so thankful for the friends Hannah had throughout elementary school, as well as her current friends who appreciate and accept her for who she is. This has not always been easy. During her elementary years,

I would invite kids over whose parents were good friends of mine or kids that I had heard were helpful to Hannah in the classroom. Their parents encouraged their children to also include Hannah in their own playdates and birthday parties. Those kids now have a very special relationship with Hannah. They can still be counted on to always show up to support her—so important given how Hannah struggled with fitting in and making new friends not too long ago.

Although Hannah can still be socially awkward at times, her receptive and expressive language that people normally tap into when making and keeping friends has greatly improved. She is no longer bewildered by small talk. Every once in a while, I still hear her incorrectly use a word or phrase out of context (idiosyncratic speech), but she's trying to insert herself in the conversation. For her twelfth birthday, Hannah actually made her own list of friends that would be invited—a huge step.

As recently as a year ago, Hannah's main strategy for connecting with people was to share exciting facts on topics of interest to her. She would share these facts right after meeting someone because she didn't know what else to say. When the other child would share their interests, Hannah struggled to process and appreciate their input, because she was still thinking about her topic. After processing, she would have to think how to respond appropriately and immediately to the information—she worked hard trying to engage, but all she really wanted was to talk more about her preferred topic. Although she still talks a lot about cats and continually has to think of what to say, as she matures, interactions are becoming easier, more engaging, and more natural. Hannah now understands that communication is a two-way street.

Until sixth grade, Hannah was unbelievably naïve, and uninterested in concerts, social media, and most television shows. The television shows she did care for were shows targeted for a younger audience. Hannah liked them because they were simpler. It was difficult for her to connect with her peers. She would become territorial over the friends she did make, almost idolizing and suffocating them. As a result, most of her friendships didn't last long. People got close, and Hannah wore them down. It was hard for me not to be overprotective.

After a friendship ended, I wanted to call the girl's mother, apologize for Hannah, and ask the mother to persuade her daughter to give the friendship another try. Of course I didn't make that call. So, in the end, Hannah and I were disappointed and upset about the lost friendship together, but we couldn't change what had happened. In his book, *Be Different*, Robison said, "There was a time when I saw relationships as all-or-nothing. Today I recognize that I can have degrees of friendship and connection with people." I see so much of John Elder Robison in my daughter. Once again, we must learn from those that walked the journey of autism before us to understand our own children.

We continually work on the skill of responding to what other people say. Hannah admits that she still feels awkward and ridiculous in some social situations; it's easier to sit alone and read a book or play on her iPad. I try to intervene when possible to keep this from happening, so she can keep trying, keep practicing interpersonal communication skills, and keep making new friends. She frequently will also apologize with "sorry" when someone explains what they were trying to say. I explain to her that she doesn't need to apologize. Dr. Barry Prizant says, "Aware of their difficulty, many children apologize for themselves, almost habitually—even without understanding what they're apologizing for." I do want Hannah to be able to have meaningful relationships with others, so I encourage her to keep trying.

When Hannah has friends over, I try to schedule the activity so Connor is at his dad's place because Hannah gets so anxious, she argues with Connor as an avoidance technique. I once took Hannah, a friend, and Connor on a trip to the zoo. Hannah spent 95 percent of the time following her brother and instigating fights so she wouldn't have to deal with the bigger issue of being unable to carry on a conversation with her friend. Diversion was her way of self-preservation.

During the last school year, Hannah also found that some of her friends that she would hang out with at school were not necessarily the friends that she would have a lot in common with outside of school. My daughter was able to understand her situation and feelings and verbalize her thoughts to ask for advice. She was learning!

HOW CAN I BE A FRIEND TO SOMEONE WITH AUTISM?[29]

- Accept your friend's differences.
- Know that some kids with autism are really smart, just in a different way.
- Protect your friend from things that bother him or her.
- Talk in small sentences with simple words and use simple gestures like pointing.
- Use pictures or write down what you want to say to help your friend understand.
- Join your friend in activities that interest him or her.
- Be patient—understand that your friend doesn't mean to bother you or others.
- Wait—give him or her extra time to answer your question or complete an activity.
- Invite your friend to play with you and join you in group activities. Teach your friend how to play by showing him or her what to do in an activity or game.
- Sit near your friend whenever you can, and help him or her do things if they want you to.
- Never be afraid to ask your teacher questions about your classmates with autism.
- Help other kids learn about autism.

FOUNDATIONAL TRAINING

Executive functioning is a set of mental skills that helps a person get things done. These skills are controlled by an area of the brain known as the frontal lobe, and individuals with Asperger's syndrome struggle with these mental skills—to the point in which it almost disables them. Hannah's shaky executive functioning affects her ability to organize and plan large tasks such as school projects, develop a sense of time, adapt to surroundings, verbalize emotions, navigate transitions, utilize **working memory**, and understand others' feedback to incorporate it into her own work. Identifying these problems and the cause has allowed us to put several coping skills (tools) in place like lists, visual schedules, timers, and "chunking" projects to build Hannah's resilience.

To spew off a verbal list of tasks I want Hannah to accomplish absolutely confounds her. After giving multiple cues, she only hears the principal one. I avoid long strings of verbal instructions. Recently, when locating a new address using the navigation system in my vehicle, I asked her to repeat the directions. She echoed the complete opposite direction that she heard. "Turn left on Walnut Street," was echoed back as, "Turn right on Walnut Street." Although she has an amazing memory for written lists, she does not possess the "file cabinet" necessary to store verbal sequences—it sounds like garbled noise. I believe it's like hearing Charlie Brown's teacher speak, only considerably faster. Hannah needs time and cues. She probably won't be someone who can multi-task; instead, I offer time-order words like first, then, next, and finally to help her sequence jobs. With that level of instruction, she gets things done, but she needs adults to empower her. Parental input offers foundational training. Give those techniques a try.

Hannah didn't always understand the social and health implications of not taking care of herself, but her self-care skills are improving. I explained to her that how others see our hygiene affects our lives. Personal hygiene must be nonnegotiable. She needed help with the steps. Sequencing. She had to remember the steps and which step needs to be done first, second, third, and so on. In addition, she had to engage motor planning for each of the steps. This doesn't even account for the sensory challenges involved with each of the tasks.

Now that she's twelve, she picks out her own clothes, takes a shower, and dresses herself. A written schedule still hangs from her bathroom cabinet and serves as a crutch—all the work of her therapists. Sometimes she still leaves tangles in her hair and plaque on her teeth—mostly due to proprioception challenges. It would just be easier and faster for me to do everything for Hannah—sometimes I'm tempted to set out the clothes and brush her teeth for her like I did for years—but that would only hurt her in the long run. In fact, there's a term for that—**learned helplessness**. I want Hannah to be confident and independent, not helpless. She will only learn this from the experience of helping herself instead of depending on others. Encourage daily living skills as early as possible. (Note: I still go over her teeth a second time to alleviate unwanted costly and time-consuming dental procedures.)

I also encourage you to assign simple chores to your children and then gradually increase their complexity. We want our children to become as autonomous as possible. We aren't doing them a favor by not helping them to be what they can be. Eleanor Roosevelt said, "The surest way to make life hard for your child is to make it too easy."

EATING AVERSIONS

Hannah still does not like the feel of food in her mouth. She hates to have to chew and admits she rarely feels the sense of hunger. She can chew on a piece of steak or pork chop for five full minutes before I finally allow her to get rid of it. Her diet still mainly consists of peanut butter and jelly sandwiches, applesauce, bananas, fruit snacks, macaroni and cheese, cereal bars, spaghetti, chicken nuggets, oatmeal, ravioli, and yogurt. She prefers the same food presented in the same way, day after day. I have basically packed the same lunch for her every day since kindergarten—that's 1,260 days! The few times I try to "mix it up," the meal returns home uneaten. This is Hannah's way of asserting control—she knows her meal is safe because it's predictable.

This limited diet has led to extreme teeth issues. The food Hannah does eat tends to stick to her teeth, causing cavities. With her oral sensory challenges, we once had to take her in as a surgery patient to an ambulatory care facility to have her cavities filled. Her dentist says that not far in the future she may need root canals. Hannah does brush her own teeth in the morning, after lunch at school, and before bed, but I go back over them at home. We also make sure to visit the dentist for cleanings more frequently than the recommended six months.

FAMILY INTERACTION

Hannah is an absolute genius in the art of argument—most often with me. William Shakespeare said it best: "And though she be but little, she is fierce."[30] Hannah says, "I yell at you the most because you are the one that really listens and understands me." Hans Asperger believed that parents of kids with Asperger's should never get into an argument with them because the kids will defend or argue their idea without end. After years of disagreements and discontent, I have to agree with his advice. Though I want to avoid arguments, I do try to make Hannah understand that she needs to show respect to adults, and arguing is disrespectful. Notice the word try, as she is hardwired to speak her mind when she disagrees and smart enough to win every time. I do feel guilty when I yell at her, but the frustration is just so real.

Most of the time when Hannah engages an argument, it's because she's having a hard time understanding what she's supposed to be doing, and she's exhausted from wearing her "game face" at school. When it's time to tackle math homework, she frequently breaks down. She believes she should either already know how to solve the problem because everyone has repeatedly told her how smart she is, or she doesn't want to just follow the algorithm (that is, the process) to solve the problem—but truly wants to understand "why" that algorithm works and at 100 percent. As a math teacher, I applaud the second trait of wanting to understand the chosen process. I struggle to help her understand "why" a process is used. Confused, she'll stop, refuse to move on, and homework can take what feels like hours and ends in exhaustion.

It took a long time for me to learn that it did not help to yell, correct, or use sarcasm with her during one of these meltdowns. Instead, I use a low, slow tone and pace to help her recover. I've also provided a chart of five-minute preferred cooldowns to calm anxiety—all she has to do is choose one. These are approaches that give children with autism the structure they need to self-correct.

Once, when I had had enough, I commented during a meltdown, "Hannah, that is not pretty!"

"Of course it is not pretty," she said through the heaving tears. "I am crying and upset, Mom."

I've also learned that when Hannah is sharing a feeling, it doesn't help to come back to her with facts—it only makes the situation worse.

Her behavioral management specialist is making great strides with giving Hannah tools to calm her anxiety and practice patience with specific triggers—namely **cognitive behavioral therapy (CBT)**. CBT can be helpful in changing how a person on the spectrum thinks about and responds to feelings such as anger, sadness, or anxiety. Anxiety remains Hannah's nemesis. Autistic behaviors do serve a real purpose—if parents discover that purpose, they can help their child communicate and manage emotions. I look forward to the day when she has greater resilience solving math problems. Until she has full control over her anxiety, I'll try to face rigid and tense times with compassion and grace.

SELF-ADVOCACY

Hannah is learning to self-advocate. Self-advocacy means speaking up to help others understand what you need to be successful. At school she confidently asks questions when she does not understand. She practices maybe a little too much sometimes, though, because her teachers have learned to limit her countless "whys." Stephen Shore said that self-advocacy simply means being lost and asking for directions.

Hannah acknowledges she still has some difficulty socializing, but doesn't always understand that remarks made about her by other kids are not meant to be mean-spirited. In her mind, it's never okay to laugh at yourself when others are finding humor in something you've done. She takes it personally. She relies on the old adage: *Something is only funny if we both think it's funny, and I'm not laughing.*

While shutting off our computer the other evening, I found that Hannah had searched for "good comebacks for kids." Near the computer were her notes. It shook me, but I realized she's understanding her problems better and better, and the more she understands, the more actively she tries to help herself. Again, her knowing she has autism with all its strengths and weaknesses enables her to realize there are areas in which she must trust others' advice and put the advice into action. I hate seeing Hannah have to face daily challenges, yet watching her assertively engage coping mechanisms on her own proves she's getting stronger and more discerning. I believe building her self-awareness will empower her to reach her highest potential. In the meantime, I'll continue to reinforce that others are *laughing with her* and not *laughing at her*, but we know how well that usually goes.

To anyone who doesn't know Hannah, she may seem like a pessimist. It's not true. I'd say she's more like a survivor—a theoretical troubleshooter. In stressful situations, she'll plan for the worst outcome. Then, she's happy because the outcome isn't nearly as bad as she had assumed—she's definitely not experiencing Psychology 101's self-fulfilling prophecy. At age ten, I asked Hannah if she wanted to compete in our local oratorical contest, which always selects a theme related to the benefits of being an optimist. Hannah's first question was, "Mom, you really think I'm an optimist?"

"Yes, absolutely."

Hannah looks at ways to make the world a better place. With that comes the realization that difficult problems are keeping the world from becoming better, and she wants to discuss those problems. It sounds like a negative view of the world, focusing on what to fix—others may view her that way, but I disagree. It doesn't make her a pessimist at all—having the foresight to bring potential challenges to the table in hopes of solving or circumventing them seems far more optimistic than a pie-eyed dreamer who has a concrete action plan that doesn't include or address the potential pitfalls.

INTERESTS AND GIFTS

I've talked throughout this book about the importance of tapping into interests, passions, perseverations, and hobbies. As I share some of Hannah's and how we leveraged those to engage with her and explore as possible long-term investments, perhaps you'll see glimpses of what captures your own child's attention.

CAT GIRL

At age twelve, Hannah's strongest passion is animals—especially cats. Cats don't talk or ask anything of her, and I believe Hannah identifies with many of their personality traits—she's fussy about what she eats, enjoys items over people for comfort, likes to be near those she loves but doesn't want them to hold her, has heightened senses, small things fascinate her for hours, and daily rituals comfort her. She's gone through stages when she wanted to meow like a cat, draw cats obsessively, and live in a world with only cats. When Hannah is at her father's house and I ask about her day, she insists on discussing the most interesting animal fact she's come across. Sunday afternoons she volunteers at our local Humane Society, proudly introducing prospective pet owners to the animals and sharing more facts on each of them than expected. For *Genius Hour* this year, Hannah wrote her own informational text on animals that was comprehensive and completely accurate. She dreams of becoming a veterinarian, and that may end up being a great fit. Hannah's favorite series of books, *Warriors*, written by Erin Hunter, follows the adventures of four clans of wild cats. Hannah likes how the rules are spelled out for the cat clans in a specific "Warrior Code: The Principles a Warrior Must Live By." No hidden curriculum there. It is also easy to see why one of her favorite books on autism is *All Cats Have Asperger Syndrome*. I believe that while this behavior may be seen as quirky now, later its eccentricity will lead to success.

ART

I find it fitting that Hans Asperger said, "For success in science and art, a dash of autism is essential."[31] Hannah approaches sketching and painting with her own unique perspective. Her teachers tell me she refuses to use visuals of the objects she is creating; she relies solely on her memory. This works because Hannah sees life as a series of pictures, tapping the visual part of her brain to compensate for language processing. Her perspective, sense of value, and form are breathtaking. The way Hannah sees the world is a gift different from anyone else. Published composer, visual artist, and adult with autism Sarah Vaughn writes, "When there are no words for all that is in you, and you feel something has to come out, ART happens."[32] Hannah cherishes her evening art class and proudly displays her work around our home. Her pieces have won awards and have been displayed in the Indiana State Museum, the Hilbert Circle Theatre, and the office where she attended elementary school.

WRITING

Hannah's talent for writing is also exceptional. In the beginning I thought, "Where is she getting this stuff?" When I questioned her fifth grade teacher, she only laughed and said, "It's her, Lori. It's all her."

Writing is one of her **splinter skills**—strengths that may be out of propor-
tion to her other skills. While I question Hannah's receptive and expressive language, she has no trouble displaying written expressive language
in her High Ability writing class. Writing seems to allow Hannah time
to process the ambiguity of the topic or question and motor plan her
thoughts (response), whereas verbal communication requires immediate response, with no pause, no time for mapping out a response. Other
students are encouraged to "share" their papers online with Hannah so
she can comment and make corrections. Hannah uses vocabulary in her
writing she doesn't use verbally, so I periodically question her, "Where
did you get that word?" She's quick to come back with the book in
which it can be found and the context surrounding the word. We must
exploit our children's strengths and accommodate their deficits.

PIANO

Hannah also plays concert piano. She started at the age of three, but
not because she's a savant. She is not. She's always enjoyed music, from
her early Baby Einstein DVDs—Baby Bach, Baby Beethoven, and Baby
Mozart. I realized the positive effect music had on her, so at age three,
when she was still nonverbal, I found a piano teacher willing to take
her as a student. Ronda was kind enough to research best methods to
instruct music students with autism. Stephen Shore, author of *Beyond
the Wall*, says, "There are many benefits to using music with people
on the autism spectrum. One of these benefits is that music provides
the structural regularity that children with autism need. Within that
structure it is possible to expand that child's repertoire of functioning."

Only recently has Ronda revealed to me that the beginning was
full of challenges for her as well. Hannah can be somewhat of a per-
fectionist. Reading two staffs at once while working her way through
a piece for the first time frustrated Hannah. Up until a few years ago,
she expected to play it perfectly the first time through. She believed
she should have been able to instantly make fluid connections between
the treble and bass clef note positions of a new piece of music. She
thought tiny mistakes were massive problems—as if Heaven and Earth
had been turned upside down. Then she'd yell at me. She would beat on
the piano's keys with her fists while making a stern, aggravated growl.

Overwhelmed, she didn't have the words or tools to express how she felt. Sometimes it's the skill we've worked the hardest on, resilience, that she loses the most under stress. Now, she has learned replacement behaviors/skills, instead of harmful ones, for anxiety-producing stimuli. She also refers to her chart of five-minute preferred cooldowns.

Years after those first lessons, Hannah has made great strides with handling anxiety while sight-reading new pieces of music. Ronda and I continue to use coping strategies with her to lessen anxiety. Although Hannah now likes to sight-read music, she really enjoys listening to music and then trying to reproduce it on her own by ear. When she's relaxing at home, I often hear music pouring out of the office, where Hannah is playing her own serious, melancholy composition—freed from being tied to someone else's notes on a page.

SPORTS

Hannah has always struggled with team sports, but she doesn't mind participating in individual sports if it doesn't require much socializing or understanding others' actions. Aquatic therapy from the age of three to six made her a brilliant swimmer. She tired of it, though, so we looked for other ideas. She has now run cross country for two years and enjoys it. I hope it lasts, because we have fun participating in races together.

TIPS ON MAKING FRIENDS FOR CHILDREN ON THE SPECTRUM[33]

- Make sure your child knows what defines a friend.
- Therapy and early intervention for your child are key. Therapists will help guide your child with the scripted words to initiate potential peer friendships.
- If it is their least restrictive environment, place your child in a mainstreamed program in elementary school.
- Make sure the children in your child's potential friendship pool are familiar with what autism is.
- Don't underestimate the empathy of your child's peers.
- Invite your child's classmates to your home. It helps if they have similar interests.

EMERGENCIES AND ACTUAL EMERGENCIES

Hannah's emergencies aren't other people's emergencies. And if I'm in the middle of an emergency myself, I have to acquiesce to her emergency, or she won't let it go. She is notorious for **catastrophizing**. A level-two emergency can escalate to a level-ten emergency in no time flat. And while the adrenaline of those level-ten emergencies may wane, she does not forget them. Flashbacks to those situations still elicit tears.

For example, when Hannah was two years old, I accidentally left her stuffed animal in the bathroom of our local children's museum. I went back five minutes later, and the animal was gone. I tried everything I could to get that animal back and to make her forget the animal. At age twelve, Hannah still brings it up. She simply can't let it go. Every time we visit the museum, she insists on checking on the animal at the Member Services Desk. Unfortunately, over time, this experience became a sad, emotional memory for Hannah. Other situations she deems level-ten emergencies include a wanted library book that has already been checked out, a missing piece to a board game, and not being first in line. To help with this, Hannah's behavioral specialist and I made categories with level-one to level-ten headings. We had Hannah list problems she deemed were emergencies and we added our own. Next, we added appropriate reactions and feelings related to each level. Hannah was then responsible for placing each emergency into its correct category. This helped Hannah conceptualize the different reactions possible to something going wrong. We also did the same thing with the levels of friendship. This activity helped to lower Hannah's anxiety and my frustration, and also led to progress socially.

AUTISM IS A CONDITION, NOT A LABEL

I have never taken—nor will I ever take—the position that autism defines my daughter or me as a mother. Autism is not what Hannah is all about, nor am I only a mother with a special needs daughter. I don't have the puzzle-piece bumper sticker on my car or the pin on my shirt—although I could. I don't want to lose sight of the fact that I'm also a mother to an amazing boy and a passionate teacher who loves her job. Don't allow autism to be your everything.

And Hannah? I want Hannah to define herself. Autism is often defined as a disability, but I never want her to embrace such a low expectation. I don't allow the language of victimhood into our vocabulary. Instead, we use empowering words so she understands she is without limits. I have always expected more from Hannah, and I believe that has led to the positive result of achieving more success and emerging from limiting challenges. Hannah loves riding bikes, sketching animals, writing fanfiction, eating peanut butter and jelly sandwiches, swimming, and basking in the sun as it warms her face. Many things define my daughter.

We aren't in denial, though. Autism results in countless frustrations. Some people might even think Hannah is spoiled with attention, but they simply don't understand how challenged she can be.

Autism, when paired with Hannah's strong will, stubbornness, and headstrong personality, is a 24/7 reality in our lives. There is no day off with autism, and sometimes it gets the best of me. I wouldn't earn a perfect score in handling Hannah's challenges, but nobody does.

Connor knows I try to make everything seem normal, but we both know it's not. He says that he constantly feels as if he's walking on eggshells. Connor tolerates a lot of unpleasant behaviors and time-consuming activities associated with Hannah, and sometimes I forget how truly hard it must be on him. He knows this is how it has to be with her, how she sometimes focuses only on herself, and it seems as if she is at the center of her own universe. I am not the only person in my home, besides Hannah, that lives with autism; Connor does too. Our life together may not always be happy, but there is enough love for everyone.

It *is* hard, and I am proud of my son.

Life is more challenging for Hannah, but we don't allow her autism to hold us back. I want to enjoy a range of activities with both of my children. One time we tried to participate in an aboveground, extreme obstacle course. While in line, an employee announced that the excursion fifteen people ahead of us had room for a party of three. I quickly volunteered our family and told the kids we needed to go up to be fitted into our safety harnesses. Hannah absolutely would not pass the people in line. She said that it's against the rules to cut in a line of people. She insisted that this rule could not be broken. After much cajoling from me and screaming from her, she finally followed.

I can never predict how she'll respond to an activity or outing. Hannah's school autism consultant says it best: "Sometimes we just have to build the plane while it's flying."

RECOGNITION

We do countless things for our children with autism that they will never recognize. But that's okay, because the most important thing for us is to see them experience success. Their success encourages us to continue working behind the scenes. Part of the reason why autism is so hard for parents is that our children struggle to identify with us. Every once in a while, though, our children recognize our efforts—what a feeling! Not only is it nice to be thanked, but even more importantly, our children are tapping into genuine empathy. After completing this manuscript, I told Hannah that I had shared it with an accomplished author. For two days in a row, on our way home from school, she would inquire about the author's opinion of my manuscript. I would tell her that I hadn't heard. On the third day, I told her that the author had contacted me and shared that my work has the possibility of making a difference to a lot of other parents with children on the spectrum.

"Oh thank goodness, Mom! I know how much *Dragonfly* means to you! My prayers have come true."

Astonished, I had to swipe away the tears.

"Mom," she continued, "that wouldn't happen to be liquid pride running down your face, would it?"

"Well, Hannah, it sure is."

But my pride is not in the manuscript. It's in that girl. Believe me, our children may not always show it, but they love us! Motivation from Hannah means exponential effort from me. Your child will do the same. Sometimes it's just a look or a simple thumbs-up, but you'll know.

I've caught Hannah numerous times singing Christina Perri's song "Human." For a little girl who used to have trouble understanding emotion and expression, it seems clear she's expressing frustration through the words of the song that talk about biting our tongues and holding our breath, and even faking smiles. The song talks about crashing and breaking down from the words spoken by others—words like knives to the heart. Hannah has autism, but she's human. Fully alive, full of feelings—fully human. In fact, given the autism, she is uniquely human.

Most recently, as Hannah has grown older and more mature, I have had to stop speaking to others about her challenges when she is near—her feelings get hurt. I often speak on Hannah's behalf, as her advocate, but I always remember she has a mind of her own and may not agree with me. I can already see this shifting as she matures and forms her own opinions about herself. Also, I have never spoken about autism as a tangible entity separate from Hannah—one she needs to shed. It's part of who she is and helps Hannah accept herself.

Here and now, I have a daughter who has achieved insurmountable success, although the journey has been bumpy, painful, scary, and exhausting. Hannah wants to fit in with society without shedding the characteristic traits that may not define her, but play a role in every move she makes.

REFLECTION

On a warm summer afternoon, I sit at a picnic table beside the water that only two years earlier Hannah had named the Dragonfly Pond. Hannah, my nature-lover, is standing on the bridge overlooking the water, peering down at her reflection. Connor has already climbed the hill to romp on the enormous playset. The water is clearer than it was years ago—as is my vision for Hannah. She has indeed emerged, though she's not "cured" or in "recovery" as had been my vision since her tender age of eighteen months.

Hannah catches sight of a dragonfly. Its double set of wings propels the insect backward and then forward—how apropos. She follows it with her eyes and then shuffles across the bridge to get a better view. The dragonfly's iridescent wings mark its individual, accentuating dynamic. Like, Hannah, it has emerged, always carrying with it the original form and yet transformed. The creature begins to navigate an unfamiliar world that sometimes doesn't make sense. Hannah will always carry autism with her, but she has wings to fly.

What lies in Hannah's future? Only she can decide, although I feel as if my history benefited her future. Until then, I will do my best to guide her to be as independent as possible. She will continue to learn strategies and coping mechanisms to help with her struggles—while never losing the essence or the very core of who she is. While autism plays a role or manipulates that, it is not what defines her.

❧ Wisdom from the Round Table ❧

Lori R.: An expert once told me that we were wearing Cameron and ourselves out trying to make sure he was in *our world* all of the time. They explained that sometimes we needed to let Cameron have time to be autistic which, in turn, would afford our family a break.

Jen: I have never allowed disrespectful behaviors out of Noah that are not tolerated with typical kids. Autism was not going to be an excuse.

Lori V.: Logic will tell you one thing, and emotions will tell you another. That's okay. Self-doubt and anger will creep in from time to time. And that is okay, too.

Susan: Tyler is twenty-three years old and has cognitive challenges with behavior issues, and because of this he needs care 24/7. He's not toilet-trained and can't take a shower or brush his own teeth. So, yes, autism did define our life until we moved him into a residential home. However, if his behavior challenges would improve, we'd give anything to have him back in our home again.

Karen: Autism sucked the joy out of our family for a long time, and we had to reclaim that. We had to reach a point of accepting and even embracing autism before our family regained some of the happiness autism had stolen from us.

Sarah: Our dreams for Mitchell's future aren't gone; they were just the wrong dreams. Mitchell still has a future. It's just not what we thought it was.

CHAPTER FOURTEEN

a new day

Autism does not define me, nor do I define autism. My mother has taught me most everything I know how to do, and the struggle within our journey has been real. *Dragonfly* should hold mothers' hands and encourage them with hope. That's why I allow my story to be told. There is indeed hope for each individual with autism. I am proof.

—Hannah Taylor

May 2017
Hannah and I arrive at the Indiana State Fairgrounds around 1:00 to attend the Central Indiana Autism Expo. The event will highlight services, programs, resources, and supports for those affected by autism. This is the first time Hannah's attended an autism event of this magnitude, and I'm anxious to see her reaction. While Hannah now embraces her autism, I've never tried to cajole her into advocacy at large. However, at twelve years of age, I believe today will be a unique opportunity for her to tag along with me.

After entering the gate, we pay for parking and are told that the autism event is being held inside the Harvest Pavilion. We follow the winding dirt path and are directed to pull into a spot right in the middle of the fairgrounds. Since Hannah and I have no idea which building in the far distance is Harvest Pavilion, we opt to take a small courtesy bus that is making its rounds. Once inside the vehicle, two older men in the seat behind us decide to be funny and pull Hannah's long braid. She snaps her head around in preparation to give someone a piece of her mind and sees the men. She smiles at them and then laughs at their silly prank. Following a bumpy ride, we see the signage for Harvest Pavilion and are quick to jump out of our seats—happy that neither of us feels nauseated.

We enter and immediately are drawn to the sponsor's information counter full of interesting items—the Autism Society of Indiana has set out children's trade books, sponsor shirts, membership information, and resource books. Hannah quickly grabs a children's book with a zebra on the front entitled All My Stripes: A Story for Children with Autism *by Shaina Rudolph and Danielle Royer. She reads the book while I'm scanning other items and asks me if we can buy it. We purchase the book and two matching gray T-shirts with* Autism Strong *in lime green lettering before moving to the next vendor's booth.*

Instantly I spot the Meaningful Day Services *sign, and I am glad we'll get a chance to share how pleased we are with Hannah's Medicaid waiver behavioral therapist, Kait, who is contracted out of their office. We approach the counter and I say, "Hi! My name is Lori Taylor, and this is my daughter, Hannah. Hannah has Asperger's syndrome and is on Kait's caseload. We just want you to know how happy we are with her work."*

Hannah moans, "Mom!" I look at her face—her eyes plead with me to stop talking.

I excuse the both of us while she pulls me aside. "Mom, please allow me to speak for myself. I wanted to talk to them about my autism and the ways that Kait has helped me time and time again. I do have my own voice. You know what? You continue around the expo the way we're going, and I'll continue the other way and have my own experience. Then, we'll be sure to meet up in the middle."

I allow her to go. She doesn't want to experience this community together; she wants her own identity within. I believe I have my answer as to her ownership, voice, and advocacy when autism is concerned. Approximately every three booths, I step away to eye her from across the pavilion. She doesn't know I'm doing this. Her interactions appear fruitful as I see a man from a sensory therapy booth hand her a sensory gadget—she plays with it awhile and then slips it into her bag and moves to the next booth. My daughter just scored a free tool! How does she do it?

Later, we meet halfway around the expo just as she predicted, and she's excited to introduce me to the vendors she's met. First, she escorts me to the therapy dogs, and Hannah is quick to make introductions. It's obvious Hannah made a good impression all by herself. Then we're off to the sensory therapy tools, and the vendors explain that Hannah has already told them that I use many of the ones on display in my classroom. Hannah then pulls the sensory gadget out of her bag that I spied earlier and shows me how it works. Next, she pulls me toward the Indiana Resource Center for Autism's table. This vendor caught Hannah's eye because of its connection to Indiana University, my alma mater—Hannah recognized the college emblem. As I glance at the woman's nametag, I see it's Marci Wheeler. I know the name. She's published many articles on autism that I've added to my resources at home. I speak with her about her article on siblings and discuss our visit to their center when Hannah was only two years old and newly diagnosed.

As we leave the expo, I share with Hannah how proud I am of her. I ask her if we should catch the courtesy bus back to the fairground's parking lot.

"No, Mom. I have an excellent memory due to my autism, and I'll show you right where it is."

We live in a world now that encourages possibility for people with autism—we can accentuate the strengths it brings and underscore its challenges. Autism doesn't make our children less; nor does it make them more. When I asked Hannah how she scored a complimentary sensory gadget, she responded, "I guess I just have a way with people." This is anecdotal evidence that our children's lives represent opportunities—promise, not doom!

We can dream big in a society that has opened up a place for people like Hannah. During the summer of 2017, Hannah, my mother, and I traveled to Milwaukee for the Autism Society of America's national conference. During Kerry Magro's (award winning national speaker, bestselling author, and adult with autism) breakout session on bullying, a mother asked a question but prefaced it by saying, "My son was recently diagnosed with autism, but he doesn't look like he has autism."

Hannah whipped her head around and corrected, "Autism doesn't have a look." Hannah has emerged as an empowered young woman; I don't need to be so vigilant about her every interaction, because she's capable and brave enough to use her voice to advocate for herself. An incredibly smart, unique, determined, vivacious young lady with autism has changed my world. She has illuminated my experience of autism from the inside out. Everything I've done for Hannah—every appointment, every therapy, every intervention, as well as every smile, hug, and conversation—has made a difference. Your efforts will do the same for your child.

As far as I know, Hannah has never been a victim of bullying in the way that Kerry Magro described; however, I know for certain that this happens frequently in the autism community. Kerry's advice was brilliant. He said that the biggest defense to a bully is a friend that stands up for the victim and says, "This isn't okay!" Great advice, Kerry!

UNDERSTANDING THE PAST

Over this last year, I have revisited the past to process how the last decade unfolded, because at times, the fractured memories were only a blur. The maelstrom of movement required to help Hannah was beyond belief. I wouldn't have been able to share my testimony if I hadn't gone through the test of raising a child on the spectrum when everything about me was thrown off balance.

There were times when I almost lost my patience with Hannah because of autism. But I would remember that she didn't choose autism, autism chose her. I found that there was no road map or secret recipe to lead us through our journey. Patience was Hannah's gift to me. Parents of children with autism face overwhelming joy and sadness, intense love and frustration, and breathtaking wonder and fear—often within the course of a single day. Hear this. I know you're tired. I know you're physically and emotionally drained. But you have to keep going. No one else loves your child the way you do. Don't allow your child to be marginalized! I know you're only one person, but you are the world to your child. Keep your eyes on the vista—stay focused on the possibilities. Autism will not always run your family.

I found that moving our challenges of the past to the written page revealed a more realistic perspective, and I saw more than I had allowed myself to process. I had built a wall around my vulnerable heart. There were so many times Hannah would yell at me and say she didn't need me, but that was when I needed to show up the most. I craved affirmation that I was a good parent—the chaos I faced wouldn't allow me to just know that I already was a good parent. My mother, aunts, and grandmother had already shown me how. I felt so many mixed feelings about continuing to work, but now I know I made the right decision. Daycare provided socialization experiences while I didn't lose an important part of my identity. I was more than just a mom with a child with autism, and so are you. Eustacia Cutler says, "You as the mother must not morph into your child and her autism or you won't exist yourself. The identity for both mother and child must not be shortchanged. If my child does not know who I am . . . then who am I?"[34] This happens all too often. Don't let it. Keep your job or find a hobby, even if you only have time to nurture it a little each day. We must allow ourselves time outside of the autism bubble. It can be an isolating life for parents—especially those of us who are extroverted by nature. Part of being a good parent is being a good role model.

HOPE AND CHANGE: THE EMERGING

During the days of early intervention, I hoped that one day I would wake up and everything would click for Hannah. Although that's not what happened, my girl gradually grew more independent. It's harder to see change when it happens in tiny, subtle shifts over a long stretch of time, but in retrospect I could follow the progress and stopped longing for a magic bullet. We have traveled many, many miles on the spectrum to get here. The girl in front of me is incredible just the way she is. Cornelia Suskind, in the movie *Life, Animated*, said of her son, Owen, "I'm going to love you so much and hold you so tight that whatever is happening will go."[35] Mrs. Suskind's words sound all too familiar. What a brilliant documentary. Sometimes we think we can make autism disappear completely, and love and persistence will win the day. It's partly right—love and persistence wins the day, but autism doesn't disappear completely. Autism sometimes does shatter the visions we have for our children, but we get new visions and see new dreams when we arrive at this better, healthier perspective. And, I wouldn't wish Hannah's autism away now if I could. Autism plays a part in what makes her astounding!

Hope goes a long way when it comes to autism—it's motivated us to try new therapies and sign up for programs and activities. Hope helps us imagine possibilities. I had to hold onto hope until I saw all that Hannah could be, and now? Hannah herself gives hope. She celebrates and embraces her individuality, exuding confidence and surprising me with self-control. Seeing her taking risks as a mature young woman, I have hope for her and for her generation. The future is going to be more than okay—she is going to be more independent than my ongoing fears that kept me awake at night wanted me to believe. Fear is the enemy. Hope is everything, and acceptance is how it happens. Allow hope to outweigh fear.

Encourage your child to cherish the person he is meant to be. After holding out hope for the best possible outcome, you will one day realize how clear it is your child is who he is. Before I know it, Hannah will be on her own journey and running her own race. I no longer wish for that crystal ball to see into Hannah's future—I can already see where she's heading, but if I couldn't, I would be at peace.

I do wish that I could slow down time, though. It's as if I can see the sand quickly falling through the hourglass. I'd appreciate more time to ensure Hannah has all the necessary life skills to be successful on her own. But wouldn't all parents? We can't allow fear to become our ideal. We must balance fear with our loved one's autonomy. Hannah knows I'll always be only a text or a call away. I also need to be the voice in her head—to look both ways before she crosses a street and to be aware of a male's intentions. Yes, I'd love to spend as much time as possible watching this lovely but complicated creature continue to emerge into a beautiful being, more shimmering and brilliant than I ever imagined. As F. Scott Fitzgerald puts it, "I love her and that's the beginning and end of everything."[36] Yes, there is hope and persistence and love, and the greatest of those is love. Love your child, and keep defining possibilities.

MY OWN EMERGENCE

I have found that the mom I was up until a year ago was the mom Hannah needed. Now, the dragonfly has spread her wings, and I no longer need to feel as though I'm on pins and needles all the time. I, too, have transformed into something more dynamic than I could have imagined—a watermark moment of transformation. During Hannah's interventions, I went from a healthy neurotic to a wounded healer. I now feel as if it's time to live a joy-filled life after struggling with life's unexpected happenings. I spent a long time isolated from the world. There is more to me than just being a mom. Still, sometimes, I need to be reminded of that. Adversity doesn't define a person—it reveals, and may even change, who she really is. Emotional pride now supersedes the arduous, fractured memories. This unexpected journey has been life's most difficult, meaningful, and rewarding accomplishment. That's why I do what I do! And you'll find you will too.

A KIND OF PILGRIMAGE

In order to fully recover from the past, I needed to revisit some of the places that had given me either great joy or pain. I started by visiting the hospital where Hannah was born. The suites are rarely empty, but as luck would have it, that day was an exception. Allowing myself time in the room where we spent the first few days of her life brought deep comfort, confirming my evolution—another time, another woman, and almost a different family.

I then journeyed to the chapel where I had shed tears after Hannah's swallow/feeding study. I stepped into spiritual sanctity, where I was able to process how far I, emotionally, and Hannah, developmentally, have traveled on our journey. Spiritually, I felt much lighter—as if I were being carried or held in someone's arms.

Then I stopped downtown at Riley Children's Hospital. I needed to trek the same route through the hospital that we had so many years ago for feeding therapy after feeding therapy. Even though this time I didn't need to worry about the automatic doors, lines on the floor, elevator buttons, or the alluring fountain, I did allow myself to look at them. Even if Hannah had been with me, there would have been no anguish because she has grown so much. I believe I wore the grin of a Cheshire cat when I discovered they had renovated the winding hallway we'd used. The tiles that aligned the passageway were painted with dragonflies. Dragonflies! I slowed and stared—I even stopped and looked closer: indigo, iridescent, gleaming. I zoomed in and snapped a quick picture with my phone. I looked down the passageway to see all the colors they'd chosen—chartreuse, rose, and apricot. And all those wings, it seemed they might each take flight at any moment and fly free. This was all I needed to see. I walked the rest of the winding hallway, turned around, retraced my steps, and went out the door, never to return.

TODAY

Hannah just finished her sixth grade year, and I learned more about her strengths and challenges by having her on our academic team. Watching her interact with others in group situations was serendipitous! We just had her middle school transition conference. As usual, I staunchly advocated for her needs. I believe I've prepared her for this next stretch. I know I can't rescue Hannah from every challenge, and she's learning to problem-solve on her own. She'll fail at times, but that's how she'll learn to manage with resilience. My hope now is no longer to seek a cure—though if someone finds one, I'll be first in line to learn more. No, my goal is that she'll practice resilience.

I've learned that no doctor or specialist can determine the limits of our children—even as parents we can't fully predict or imagine the possibilities. But we will continue to have *hope*. Nothing is predetermined and time together is filled with open-ended opportunity.

Hannah has asked me about her future and whether she will always need to disclose that she has autism. I told her that others don't go around saying they don't have autism, so of course not. But it is important that she always advocate for what she needs. Disclosure will need to be her decision. I have no doubt Hannah will experience insurmountable success—she's too stubborn to do anything else.

A JOY-FILLED LIFE

Only by looking at the past can we allow it to become the past. And the past will no longer mess with our family's today. Change happens when one hurts enough, learns enough, or receives enough. It takes a while and can be trying, but you'll get there, too. My transcendent moment came when Connor asked, "Are you happy, Mom?"

To which Hannah replied, "She cries because she's had to be strong too long."

That was when I knew that I had to do everything to get back the pride, love, and honor in the person I am. The wounded healer needed her life back. And that is just what I'm doing. No more survival—but flourishing! As I step back and look at what I've accomplished, I'm reminded I am a worthy person. I am closing the doors that caused me pain, anger, and suffering. I look forward to opening the ones that will bring me love, inner peace, and, most of all, happiness. Autism has been a huge part of my identity. I have been revolving around the autism orbit for a very long time. Hannah this . . . Autism that . . . I started with the question, "What makes me happy?" It had been such a long time since I'd thought that much about myself and my own desires, I really didn't know the answer. I set off on a journey trying to redefine myself.

My children and I live in a beautiful home that I was blessed to get an unbelievable deal on after I divorced. In all these years, I had never taken the time to hang many pictures on the walls or decorate any room but the kids' rooms. I looked at the kids' pictures that I did have up—they were covered in dust and from the year before my husband left. It was as if time had stopped. I was still living in Hannah's diagnosis and my divorce. I decided to start with the present. I set up new photo sessions, ordered prints, and hung them on the walls of the family room. I also added to the pictures on Hannah and Connor's growth charts—I was five years behind! We began projects I'd only dreamed about, like gardening. The kids and I planted our first garden the summer of 2017 and enjoyed its returns. Connor and I play more chess and he continues to outsmart me every time. We've been shooting more baskets and engineering more contraptions. Hannah and I enjoy leisurely bike rides where she takes the lead, and our daily devotional reminds us both of life's lessons. Laughter rings through the house more often than ever before. I no longer mourn our past—letting it go has brightened all of our futures. I have donated most of our therapy tools and resources, including the PECS cards and the emotions jigsaw puzzle, and thrown out many of my anecdotal records. My new, more positive outlook on life has been contagious to my children. We are making better memories and living in the present. Our home is becoming a haven. The weight has been lifted!

One day while walking into school, I told Hannah we were going to have a low-anxiety day. "Could you try to not let your autism get the best of you?"

"I'll try," she said. She paused before pulling the door open and added, "Can you also try not to let it get the best of you?"

Touché.

She and I are now both trying to embrace a joy-filled, low-anxiety life. We have our bumps in the road, but that's to be expected. It's a new day for the Taylor Trio. Choose joy for your family.

A FINAL WORD

Be your child's champion! I know it's a round-the-clock job, especially when your child is young. Remember, you're enough as you are; you won't always feel as you do today. And people aren't looking at you as the mother with a child diagnosed with autism.

Along our journey, and against insurmountable odds, something extraordinary happened to us.

I will continue to teach and advocate for those families with children on the spectrum, and I'll enjoy the future that is waiting for me and invite you to do the same. It's time to open my home more to family and friends—just one of the things that stopped over a decade ago.

Writing has been cathartic and healing—it's my forte. Although it was difficult turning our private experiences into a public manuscript, I was driven to understand a difficult time. I looked back on the woman I used to be and uncovered how I became who I am now. It was a long haul. You might try to find a way to capture your story as it unfolds in a journal or as letters to someone who will understand. I've continued to chronicle our story at my website, www.emergingfromautism.com. You can follow my blog there and explore the resources I continually collect and make available. Emerging from Autism has also become a venue for others touched by autism. Seek solace in its words and understanding.

My hope for your family is that your interventions make your child as independent as possible, your awareness spreads throughout your community, and you and your child's advocacy is one of a mighty warrior. Services for children with autism are getting better and better every single day as a result of caring individuals devoted to advocacy. Brave autism's journey while celebrating each step of progress!

THE TOP LESSONS MY DAUGHTER WITH AUTISM HAS TAUGHT ME

Being on the front lines with Hannah's autism has made me a better mom, teacher, and person—she has definitely taught me more than I could teach her in a lifetime.

* Hannah will be the first to tell you that she is different—not less or more.
* Although autism plays a significant role in Hannah's daily interactions, it does not define her.
* Not all individuals have the same sensory systems.
* Some people think literally and in pictures.
* When I tell my daughter something is going to happen, it better happen or I'm going to wish it had.
* The ticket into many of our children's worlds is their affinities.

- What I believe makes an individual happy doesn't necessarily make Hannah happy.
- What is a challenge today may not be a challenge tomorrow.
- Hannah doesn't learn by watching others. Social pragmatics need to be taught directly. When she does try to imitate the movements of others, like waving, it is difficult.
- It is imperative that I no longer discuss Hannah's challenges in front of her.
- I not only need to tell Hannah to stop doing something—I need to give her the reason why.
- Flapping (stimming) just meant that Hannah wanted to communicate.
- I cannot give Hannah a list of things to complete; they need to be broken down into steps.
- For every challenge that autism has given to Hannah, it has also given her a gift.
- Behavior is a form of communication.
- Receptive and expressive language don't always correlate with aptitude.
- Mind-blindness inhibits Hannah's ability to see things from a different viewpoint.
- I did nothing to cause Hannah's autism.
- The frontal lobe of the brain controls a set of mental skills that help to get things done—executive function—and Hannah's doesn't work as efficiently as others, so I need to be patient when things aren't done.
- Stretching children on the spectrum to appreciate new experiences takes baby steps. If stretched too far too quickly, they will break.
- It's often difficult for children with autism to navigate friendships.
- Routines and schedules play an important role for people with autism by helping to create stability and

order. Their brains must know what is coming and what to expect.

* A sensory retreat is a crucial component that assists self-regulation by helping a child on the spectrum recover from "fight or flight" and return to a ready state.

* Diagnosed with autism or not, children shouldn't always be rescued from challenges. They should be taught how to face challenges with resilience.

* A child with autism may look like he is ignoring you, but he is instead waiting for you to enter his world.

* Swinging, jumping, spinning, and rocking provide vestibular input to the brain and allow children with autism to organize their bodies and regulate their sensory systems.

* Lining up toys, crayons, or cards provides order, comfort, and a sense of control for children on the spectrum that they often lack.

* Water (aquatic therapy) is a medium that provides ideal conditions to enhance language, decrease stimming, and increase eye contact for those with autism.

* Chronological age and developmental age will most likely not be in sync for kids on the autism spectrum. There is usually asynchronous, uneven development.

* Children with autism are heavily dependent on cues and prompts in order to move on to the next task—even when they are able to identify the next task.

* Children on the spectrum tend to see the parts of an image or idea (gestalt) before the entire image or idea materializes. Stephen Shore referred to this as "central coherence" at the Autism Society of America's national conference in Milwaukee, Wisconsin in 2017. I refer to it as a bug's-eye view.

* Those with autism tend to have an innate connection with nature that provides a peaceful affect.

- Society has general rules that others learn from observation. This hidden curriculum must be directly taught to children on the spectrum.
- Acting as someone that you aren't is the highest form of self-harm and is exhausting. Allow your kids to be themselves!
- Individuals with autism are capable of feeling sympathy for others, but cognitive empathy (inferring mental state) is more of a struggle. They possess emotional valence—acuity.
- Self-advocacy for individuals with autism means they must expect people to treat them with dignity and respect while also requesting what is needed in order to succeed.
- No doctor can make a definite prognosis as to the heights that individuals with autism can achieve. Hope and early intervention are the best medicine.

Wisdom from the Round Table

Lori R.: When just beginning our autism journey, one of the best pieces of advice that I received from a mother who had been on the journey much longer was this: "However you want your family and friends to see Cameron is how you have to live." My husband and I took this to heart and made it one of our family's mottos.

Jen: Last night we set an alarm for the very last time that was labeled *school* on Noah's calendar. This morning I watched my biggest blessing step up on a school bus for the very last time. I'm so proud of Noah and all he has accomplished. I know he'll continue to smile and be that fun, loving, kindhearted man.

Lori V.: I have recently made a job change out of state, and Byron and I moved. Devin, my neurotypical son, remains in college in our hometown, which is hard for me, but I know it's best for him. Byron and I are excited about our new journey. It feels good.

Susan: Bruce and I just took our first vacation without the kids in fifteen years. As I sat at the pool, I realized just how different our life was than everyone else's. It's really hitting home how Allie grew up and how atypical our family was due to Ty's special needs.

Karen: Both of our boys with autism are now in college in different capacities. Eric lives at home and commutes, which is better for him. John is away at college and had a successful first year.

Sarah: Mitchell just completed his eighth grade year. His middle school years were more sustainable with an excellent Teacher of Record providing the supports he needs. We look forward to his growth toward independence in high school.

epilogue

**"The Life of a Dragonfly
and a Child with Autism"**
by
Hannah Grace Taylor

I am a dragonfly.
My egg is gently placed upon a leaf.
It slips into the water, slowly sinking to the bottom of the pond.
I wonder when my mother will come back.
I am stuck in the pond, with nothing to do for four years.
I cry.
I am a child with autism.
I pop out of my mom's belly and stare at the people around me.
I am taken to a house where I meet lots of people.
But, sadly, for four years I cannot talk to them.
I am captured in my own world, and I don't understand a thing.
I cry.
I am a dragonfly.
While in the pond, I slowly bubble to its surface, and am transformed.
My mother is not here.
I see trees and the sky with the sun.
What am I meant to do?
I cry.

I am a child with autism.

I see the doctor staring at me as he tells my parents something.

I am uncomfortable when someone or something touches my skin.

Why do people make me eat?

I flap my hands because the words simply aren't there.

I cry.

I am a dragonfly.

Hope rises, and I begin to reveal my concealed wings.

I propel my wings backward, and then forward.

I see other dragonflies and understand what I am meant to do.

I cry.

I am a child with autism.

I have a schedule, work with therapists, and I love, love, love cats.

I now appreciate hugs and kisses from my family.

I have begun to understand language and what I am meant to do.

I become more independent every day.

I cry with happiness.

You know I do.

I cry.

Glossary, Endnotes, Suggested Resources, and Index

glossary

affinity: A strong attachment, liking, or passion for specific items, ideas, topics, or possessions.

applied behavior analysis (ABA): A set of principles that form the basis for many behavioral treatments. ABA is based on the science of learning and behavior. This science includes general "laws" about how behavior works and how learning takes place. ABA therapy applies these laws to behavior treatments in a way to increase useful or desired behaviors. ABA also applies these laws to reduce behaviors that may interfere with learning or behaviors that may be harmful. ABA therapy is used to increase language and communication skills. It is also used to improve attention, focus, social skills, memory, and academics. ABA can be used to decrease problem behaviors.

Asperger's syndrome: One of several previously separate subtypes of autism that were folded into the single diagnosis of autism spectrum disorder (ASD) with the publication of the DSM-5. Asperger's syndrome was generally considered to be on the high-functioning end of the spectrum. Affected children and adults have difficulty with social interactions and exhibit a restricted range of interests and/or repetitive behaviors. Motor development may be delayed, leading to clumsiness or uncoordinated motor movements. Compared with those affected by other forms of ASD, however, those with Asperger's syndrome typically do not have significant delays or difficulties in language or cognitive development. Some even demonstrate precocious vocabulary—often in a highly specialized field of interest.

cognitive behavioral therapy (CBT): A form of psychotherapy that treats problems and boosts happiness by modifying dysfunctional emotions, behaviors, and thoughts.

catastrophizing: To view or talk about an event or situation as worse than it really is.

cognitive empathy: The largely conscious drive to recognize accurately and understand another's emotional state.

cognitive flexibility: The mental ability to transition between thinking about two different concepts.

***Diagnostic and Statistical Manual of Mental Disorders, Fifth Edition* (DSM-5):** The 2013 update to the American Psychiatric Association's classification and diagnostic tool.

echolalia: The repetition of words, phrases, intonation, or sounds of the speech of others.

executive functioning: A set of mental skills such as organizing, planning, sustaining attention, and inhibiting inappropriate responses.

failure to thrive: Usually defined in terms of weight, and can be evaluated either by a low weight for the child's age, or by a low rate of increase in the weight.

floortime: A therapy whose premise is that adults can help children expand their circles of communication by meeting them at their developmental level and building on their strengths. The technique challenges children to push themselves to their fullest potential. It develops "who they are," rather than "what their diagnosis says." Encourages parents to engage children literally at their level—by getting on the floor to play.

food jags: An individual will only eat one food item, or a very small group of food items, meal after meal.

hyperlexia: A syndrome characterized by a child's precocious ability to read; however, these children also exhibit extreme difficulty with oral communication, social interaction, and expression.

hidden curriculum: Refers to the unwritten, unofficial, and often unintended lessons, values, and perspectives that students learn in school.

inclusion: The concept is based on the idea that students with disabilities should not be segregated, but should be included in a classroom with their typically developing peers. A student in an inclusion classroom usually needs only to show that she is not losing out from being included in the classroom, even if she is not necessarily making any significant gains.

Individual Education Plan (IEP): The law states that each child that receives special education services must have an IEP. This important legal document spells out a child's learning needs, the services the school will provide, and how progress will be measured.

interoception: The eighth sense and responsible for detecting internal regulation responses, such as respiration, hunger, heart rate, and the need for digestive elimination.

joint attention: Two people share interest in an object or event and there is an understanding between the two people that they are both interested in the same object or event.

learned helplessness: A condition in which an individual has come to believe he or she is helpless in a situation, even when this is untrue. As it pertains to the text, a child *believes* he is unable to perform an action or skill because someone has always done it for him.

mainstreaming: The concept is based on the fact that a student with disabilities may benefit from being in a general education classroom, both academically and socially. A mainstreamed student may have slight adjustments in how she is assessed, but she learns mostly the same material and must show that she is gaining from her classroom placement.

mind-blindness: A theory that states individuals with autism are unable to form an awareness of others' thoughts. Also known as a lack of theory of mind.

midline: An imaginary line running through the middle of the body.

mirror neurons: A type of brain cell that responds equally when we perform an action and when we witness someone else perform the same action.

motor plan: A process that encompasses the ability to come up with an idea, plan how to complete the idea, and then finally, execute that idea. Children with sensory processing disorder often have difficulty motor planning for various gross motor and fine motor tasks, as motor planning is a complex procedure that relies on the efficient integration of sensory information.

oral sensory dysfunction: A symptom of sensory processing disorder in which a child's hypersensitivity may cause oral defensiveness, not allowing food or a toothbrush into the mouth. However, a hyposensitivity may cause a child to place inedible objects into their mouth.

perseveration: The repetition of a word, phrase, or gesture to an exceptional degree. Perseverative acts include object perseveration, action perseveration, and verbal perseveration.

pervasive developmental disorder (PDD): An umbrella term for a wide spectrum of disorders referred to as Autism Spectrum Disorders (ASD). The terms PDD and ASD are used interchangeably. They are a group of neurobiological disorders that affect a child's ability to interact, communicate, relate, play, imagine, and learn.

Pervasive Developmental Disorder-Not Otherwise Specified (PDD-NOS): One of several previously separate subtypes of autism that were folded into the single diagnosis of autism spectrum disorder (ASD) with the publication of the DSM-5. In the past, psychologists and psychiatrists often used the terms pervasive developmental disorders and autism spectrum disorders interchangeably. As such, PDD-NOS became the diagnosis applied to children or adults who are on the autism spectrum but do not fully meet the criteria for another ASD such as autistic disorder (sometimes called "classic" autism) or Asperger's syndrome.

Picture Exchange Communication System (PECS): A program that begins by teaching an individual to give a picture of a desired item to a "communicative partner," who immediately honors the exchange as a request. The system goes on to teach discrimination of pictures and how to put them together in sentences. In the more advanced phases, individuals are taught to answer questions and to comment.

proprioception: The relationship of one body part to another, and the relationship of the movement of a body part to the needed strength to produce an action. It allows an individual to know where their body is in space.

Rett syndrome: A rare, non-inherited genetic postnatal neurological disorder that occurs almost exclusively in girls and leads to severe impairments, affecting nearly every aspect of the child's life: their ability to speak, walk, eat, and even breathe easily.

sensory diet: a carefully designed, personalized activity plan that provides the sensory input that a person needs to feel focused and organized throughout the day.

sensory modulation: An attempt to calm or manage the reactions of adjusting to one's environment.

sensory processing disorder: A condition in which the brain has trouble receiving and responding to information that comes in through the senses. Formerly referred to as sensory integration dysfunction, it is not currently recognized as a distinct medical diagnosis.

self-regulation: An individual's ability to acknowledge and respond to internal and external sensory input, and then adjust emotions and behavior to the demands of his surroundings.

social pragmatics: Rules for using functional spoken language in a meaningful context or conversation.

Social Stories: Developed by Carol Gray in 1990, these individualized short stories depict a social situation that a child affected by autism may encounter. These stories are used to teach communal skills through the use of precise and sequential information about everyday events that a child may find difficult or confusing, thus preventing further anxiety on the part of the child.

Somatization Disorder: A mental disorder characterized by recurring, multiple, and current clinically significant complaints about anxiety. Intense thoughts, feelings, and behavior interfere with daily life.

splinter skills: A precocious, highly developed behavior or talent that occurs in isolation. One that is not associated with other cognitive or social skills.

stimming: Self-stimulating behaviors are stereotyped or repetitive movements or posturing of the body.

theory of mind: Refers to one's ability to perceive how others think and feel, and how that relates to oneself.

twice-exceptional (2e): Intellectually gifted children who have some form of disability.

vestibular: A body system that includes the middle and inner ear and gives an individual the sense of balance and movement.

video modeling: A visual teaching method that occurs by watching a video of someone modeling a targeted behavior or skill and then imitating the behavior or skill watched.

working memory: The thinking skill that focuses on memory-in-action: the ability to remember and use relevant information while in the middle of an activity.

endnotes

Chapter One: The "D" Word (Diagnosis/Identification)

1. "14 Signs of Autism." *Future Horizons* poster, 2015.
2. "Why Does My Kid Do That?: 10 Common Signs of Sensory Processing Disorder." *Sensory World* poster, 2015.

Chapter Two: Life Before Autism

3. Warner, Dr. Jason. Interview. 30 June 2017.

Chapter Three: Something's Not Quite Right

4. "Autism Screening." *Hands in Autism* handout, 2009.
5. "Autism Screening." *Hands in Autism* handout, 2009.

Chapter Four: Rewriting the Script

6. Stone, Wendy. "Early Intervention." *Autism Speaks*, www.autism-speaks.org/family-services/tool-kits/100-day-kit/early-intervention. Accessed 5 July 2017.
7. Pausch, Randy. "The Last Lecture." *Hyperion,* 2008.

Chapter Five: A Baby Boy is Born

8. Wheeler, Marci. "Sibling Perspectives: Guidelines for Parents." *Autism Society of America*, www.autism-society.org/wp-content/uploads/2014/04/sibling-perspectives.pdf. Accessed 5 July 2017.

9. Cherry, Jason. "Sibling Empowerment: A Funny Thing Happened On the Way Through Autism." Autism Society of America national conference, 2015.

10. Fialco, Dana. "Five Benefits of Growing Up With an Autistic Sibling." *Autism Speaks,* www.autismspeaks.org/node/119681. Accessed 5 July 2017.

Chapter Seven: Changing Normal

11. "Facts and Misconceptions about Autism Spectrum Disorder." *Hands in Autism* handout, 2016.

12. "Facts and Misconceptions about Autism Spectrum Disorder." *Hands in Autism* handout, 2016.

13. Suskind, Ron. "'Life, Animated': Parents Describe How Animated Characters Helped Son With Autism Connect." *Nightline,* June 2016.

Chapter Eight: Holidays and Vacations

14. Bricker, Angela. "Help! We Just Want to Take a Family Vacation!" *Autism Companion,* June 2014, p. 46.

Chapter Nine: Flying Solo

15. Bennie, Maureen. "How do I keep my marriage strong while raising a child with autism?" Autism Awareness Centre Inc., www.autismawarenesscentre.com/keep-marriage-strong-raising-child-autism. Accessed 5 July 2017.

16. Abbott, Alysia. "Love in the Time of Autism." *Psychology Today,* www.psychologytoday.com/articles/201307/love-in-the-time-autism. Accessed 5 July 2017.

17. *The Oprah Winfrey Show*. Harpo Studios, April 2007.

18. Diament, Michelle. "Autism Moms Have Stress Similar To Combat Soldiers." *Disability Scoop,* www.disabilityscoop.com/2009/11/10/autism-moms-stress/6121. Accessed 5 July 2017.

19. "Autism Support Group Meeting Clip From Parenthood." YouTube, www.youtube.com/watch?v=5go3SBU6UNM. Accessed 5 July 2017.

20. Bennie, Maureen. "How do I keep my marriage strong while raising a child with autism?" Autism Awareness Centre Inc., www.autismawarenesscentre.com/keep-marriage-strong-raising-child-autism. Accessed 5 July 2017.

Chapter Ten: Both Sides of the Table

21. Grandin, T. *The Way I See It*. Future Horizons, 2008.
22. Ginott, Haim. *Teacher and Child: A Book for Parents and Teachers*. Macmillan, 1975.
23. Lovaas, Ivar. "Quote: Dr. O. Ivar Lovaas." The Behavior Station. thebehaviorstation.com/lovaas-quote/?format=pdf. Accessed 5 July 2017.
24. Notbohm, E. *Ten Things Your Student with Autism Wishes You Knew*. Future Horizons, 2006.

Chapter Twelve: Autism Anecdotes

25. "Tips for Supporting Social Interaction." Autism Speaks, www.autismspeaks.org/sites/default/files/autism_friendly_youth_organizations.pdf. Accessed 5 July 2017.

Chapter Thirteen: Acceptance and Fostering Independence

26. O'Toole, Jennifer. *Sisterhood of the Spectrum: An Asperger Chick's Guide to Life*. Jessica Kingsley Publishers, 2015.
27. Pia. "In Their Own Words—Glows." Autism Speaks, www.autismspeaks.org/blog/2012/06/20/their-own-words-glows. Accessed 5 July 2017.
28. O'Toole, Jennifer. *Asperkids: An Insider's Guide to Loving, Understanding and Teaching Children with Asperger Syndrome*. Jessica Kingsley Publishers, 2012.
29. "How Can I Be a Friend To Someone with Autism?" Autism Society of America, handout.
30. Shakespeare, William. *A Midsummer Night's Dream*, 1595, Act 3, Scene 2.
31. Borgman, Stephen. "Here Are 10 Great Autism Spectrum Quotes." *Psychology Today*, www.psychologytoday.com/blog/spectrum-solutions/201012/here-are-10-great-autism-spectrum-quotes. Accessed 5 July 2017.
32. O'Toole, Jennifer. *Sisterhood of the Spectrum: An Asperger Chick's Guide to Life*. Jessica Kingsley Publishers, 2015.
33. Woliver, Robbie. "Autism can be your child's ally, not enemy, in making friends: 5 tips on turning peers to pals." *Psychology Today*,

www.psychologytoday.com/blog/alphabet-kids/201006/autism-can-be-your-childs-ally-not-enemy-in-making-friends-5-tips-turning. Accessed 5 July 2017.

Chapter Fourteen: A New Day

34. Cutler, Eustacia. "A Day with the great Eustacia Cutler!" Aspergers101, www.aspergers101.com/day-great-eustacia-cutler. Accessed 5 July 2017.
35. Suskind, Ron. *Life, Animated*. Motto Pictures, 2016.
36. Fitzgerald, F. Scott. *Dear Scott, Dearest Zelda: The Love Letters of F. Scott and Zelda Fitzgerald*. Bloomsbury Publishing, 2002.

suggested resources

If you, a family member, or a friend have been diagnosed with autism, I recommend the following resources: books, movies, television shows, and websites for further insight into each of the topics discussed in *Dragonfly: A Daughter's Emergence from Autism: a Practical Guide for Parents*.

Books for Children and Teens

Draper, S. (2012) *Out of My Mind*. London: Antheneum Books for Young Readers.

Ely, L. (2004) *Looking After Louis*. Morton Grove, IL: Albert Whitman and Company.

Hoopmann, K. (2006) *All Cats Have Asperger Syndrome*. London: Jessica Kingsley Publishers.

Hoopmann, K. (2013) *Inside Asperger's Looking Out*. London: Jessica Kingsley Publishers.

James, Lindsay. (2016) *The A in Autism Stands for Awesome*. Jackson, NJ: BoBo Books, LLC.

Lord, C. (2006) *Rules*. New York: Scholastic Press.

Moore-Mallinos, J., Fabrega, M. (2008) *My Brother is Autistic*. Hauppauge, New York: Barron's.

Montgomery, S. (2012) *Temple Grandin: How the Girl Who Loved Cows Embraced Autism and Changed the World*. New York: Houghton Mifflin Books for Children.

Peete, H., Peete, R. E. (2010) *My Brother Charlie*. New York: Scholastic Press.

Peralta, S., (2002) *All About My Brother*. Shawnee Mission, KS: Autism Asperger Publishing Company.

Rorby, G. (2017) *How to Speak Dolphin*. New York: Scholastic Press.

Rudolph, S., Royer, D. (2015) *All My Stripes: A Story for Children with Autism*. Washington, DC: Magination Press.

Stefanski, D. (2011) *How to Talk to an Autistic Kid*. Minneapolis, MN: Free Spirit Publishing Inc.

Thomas, Pat. (2014) *I See Things Differently: A First Look at Autism*. Hauppauge, NY: Barron's Educational Series, Inc.

Yacio, J. (2015) *Temple Did It, And I Can, Too! Seven Simple Life Rules*. Arlington, TX: Sensory World.

Books for Adults

Attwood, T., Grandin, T., Faherty, C., Wagner, S., Wrobel, M., Bolick, T., Iland, L., Myers, Jennifer., Snyder, R. (2006) *Asperger's and Girls*. Arlington, TX: Future Horizons.

Baker, J. (2001) *The Social Skills Picture Book: Teaching Communication, Play, and Emotion*. Arlington, TX: Future Horizons.

Barnett, K. (2013) *The Spark: A Mother's Story of Nurturing, Genius, and Autism*. New York: Random House.

Cariello, C. (2015) *What Color is Monday? How Autism Changed One Family for the Better*. London: Jessica Kingsley Publishers.

Carter, L. K. (2016) *Ketchup is My Favorite Vegetable: A Family Grows Up with Autism*. London: Jessica Kingsley Publishers.

Donvan, J., Zucker, C. (2016) *In A Different Key: The Story of Autism*. New York: Crown Publishers.

Fields-Meyer, A. (2011) *Following Ezra*. New York: New American Library.

Grandin, T. (2008) *The Way I See It*. Arlington, TX: Future Horizons.

Higashida, N. (2007) *The Reason I Jump*. New York: Random House.

Landa, R., Marsden, M., Burrows, N., Newmark, A. (2013) *Chicken Soup for the Soul: Raising Kids on the Spectrum*. Cos Cob, CT: Chicken Soup for the Soul Publishing, LLC.

Lyons, T., and Stagliano, K. (2015) *101 Tips for the Parents of Girls with Autism*. New York: Skyhorse Publishing.

Noonan, J. (2016) *No Map to This Country*. Boston, MA: Da Capo Press.

Notbohm, E. (2005) *Ten Things Every Child with Autism Wishes You Knew*. Arlington, TX: Future Horizons.

Notbohm, E. (2006) *Ten Things Your Student with Autism Wishes You Knew*. Arlington, TX: Future Horizons.

O'Toole, J. (2012) *Asperkids: An Insider's Guide to Loving, Understanding and Teaching Children with Asperger Syndrome*. London: Jessica Kingsley Publishers.

O'Toole, J. (2015) *Sisterhood of the Spectrum: An Asperger Chick's Guide to Life*. London: Jessica Kingsley Publishers.

O'Toole, J. (2013) *The Asperkid's Secret Book of Social Rules*. London: Jessica Kingsley Publishers.

Prizant, B. (2016) *Uniquely Human: A Different Way of Seeing Autism*. New York: Simon and Schuster.

Robison, J. (2011) *Be Different*. New York: Crown Publishing.

Senator, S. (2016) *Autism Adulthood*. New York: Skyhorse Publishing.

Shore, S. (2003) *Beyond the Wall: Personal Experiences with Autism and Asperger Syndrome*. Shawnee Mission, KS: Autism Asperger Publishing Company.

Simone, R. (2010) *Aspergirls: Empowering Females with Asperger Syndrome*. London: Jessica Kingsley Publishers.

Stagliano, K. (2010) *All I Can Handle: I'm No Mother Teresa*. New York: Skyhorse Publishing.

Movies

Extremely Loud and Incredibly Close (2011) Motion picture directed by Stephen Daldry. Warner Brothers.

Finding Dory (2016) Motion picture directed by Andrew Stanton. Pixar.

Life, Animated (2016) An independent film directed by Roger Ross Williams. The Orchard.

Rain Man (1988) Motion picture directed by Barry Levinson. United Artists.

Temple Grandin (2010) Biopic directed by Mick Jackson. HBO.

The Accountant (2016) Motion picture directed by Gavin O'Connor. Warner Brothers.

Television Shows

Atypical (2017-?) Sam Gardner performed by Keir Gilchrist.

Grey's Anatomy (2008-2009) Virginia Dixon performed by Mary McDonnell.

Parenthood (2010-2015) Max Braverman performed by Max Burkholder.

Sesame Street (2017-?) Julia performed by Stacey Gordon.

The Big Bang Theory (2007-?) Sheldon Cooper performed by Jim Parsons.

The Good Doctor (2017-?) Shaun Murphy performed by Freddie Highmore.

Websites

All websites were accessed July 5, 2017.

Asperkids—Jennifer O'Toole at www.asperkids.com.

Autism Society at www.autism-society.org.

Autism Speaks at www.autismspeaks.org.

Barry Prizant at www.barryprizant.com.

Carrie Cariello—Exploring the Colorful World of Autism at www.carriecariello.com.

John Elder Robison at www.johnrobison.com.

Kerry Magro at www.kerrymagro.com.

Liane Kupferberg Carter at www.lianekupferbergcarter.com.

Lori Ashley Taylor at www.emergingfromautism.com.

Stephen Shore at www.autismasperger.net.

Susan Senator at www.susansenator.com.

Temple Grandin at www.templegrandin.com.

index

A Thorn in My Pocket (Cutler), 96
accommodations, 22, 90, 114, 119,
    141–142, 172, 177, 182, 188, 195
Ackerman, Diane, *xxii*
affinities, 91–92, 124–125, 172,
    186, 263
All Cats Have Asperger Syndrome
    (Hoopmann), 243, 283
anecdotes, 203–221
annual case review (ACR), 109, 178
Applied Behavior Analysis (ABA),
    53, 126, 181, 273
aquatic therapy, *xxxi*, 120, 143, 207,
    245, 265
Asperger, Hans (MD), 239, 243
Asperger's syndrome, *xxiii, xxvi, xxxi,*
    91, 95, 119, 128, 185, 203, 211,
    225, 230, 237, 254, 273, 276
Asperkids (O'Toole), 95, 227,
    285–286
attention deficit hyperactivity
    disorder (ADHD), 14
autism,
    diagnosis, *xx-xxiii, xxvi-xxviii,*
        xxx-xxxi, 1–14, 22–24, 28,

        35–37, 41, 43–45, 52, 64,
        67, 80–81, 83, 85, 87, 95,
        98, 105–106, 123, 139, 142,
        150, 150, 152–155, 157,
        160, 171, 174, 188, 192,
        195, 199–200, 209, 225,
        261, 273–274, 276
    facts, 104
    misconceptions, 105
    signs, 6, 25–38
Autism Science Foundation (ASF), 13
Autism Society of America (ASA),
    56, 78, 88, 93, 113, 127, 165,
    227, 256, 265
Autism Society of Indiana (ASI), 254
Autism Speaks, 56, 87, 95, 286
autism spectrum disorder (ASD), 35,
    43, 46, 66, 70, 104–105, 131,
    170, 220, 226, 273, 276.

Baby Einstein, 30, 53, 136, 244
back-to-school, 180
Baker, Jed (PhD), 96, 103, 284
Ball, James (ED), 93
Baron-Cohen, Simon, 233

bathing, 30, 33, 50
Be Different (Robison), 178,
    230–231, 235, 285
behavior plans, 176, 184
behavioral psychologist, *xxx*, 1,8,
    11–12, 35, 44, 58
behavioral therapy, *xxxi*
Benson, Ezra Taft, 129
*Beyond the Wall: Personal
    Experiences with Autism and
    Asperger Syndrome* (Shore), 93,
    244, 285
blogs, 93–95, 98
Bloom (Hampton), 93
Burns, Michele Pierce, 153

Campbell, Joseph, *xxiv*, 223
Cariello, Carrie, 95, 284, 286
Carter, Liane Kupferberg, 67, 154,
    284, 286
case conferences, 109, 114, 116,
    170–173, 178–179
catastrophizing, 246, 274
Centers for Disease Control
    (CDC), *xxi*
Cherry, Cathy Purple, 165
Cherry, Jason, 78
CNN Headline News, *xx*
Coelho, S. L., 1
cognitive empathy, 75, 211, 266, 274
cognitive flexibility, 143, 274
Collins, Paul, 228
Cummings, Conner, 90
Cummings, Sharon, 90
Cutler, Eustacia, 36, 96, 257
Daniels, Braden, 84

denial, *xxiii*, 35–36, 43, 247

developmental pediatrician, *xxx*, 9,
    35, 57
developmental preschool, *xxxi*, 101,
    105–106, 112, 114, 120, 171,
    176, 187, 196
developmental therapy, *xxx*, 3, 44,
    49, 55, 151
Devine, Adele, 25
*Diagnostic and Statistical Manual of
    Mental Disorders, Fifth Edition
    (DSM-5)*, *xi*, 119, 203, 273–274,
    276
dietitian, *xxx*, 57
divorce, 129, 150, 152–153,
    161–162, 192–193, 197–198,
    261
Donvan, John, 83, 93, 284

early intervention, *xxii-xxiii, xxix-
    xxx,* 35–36, 39–61, 101–128,
    157, 160, 176, 195, 200, 245,
    257, 266
*Early Intervention and Autism:
    Real-Life Answers, Real-Life
    Questions* (Ball), 93
Early Intervention Programs, 35
echolalia, 113, 172, 274
education, *xxi, xxvi, xxvii*, 9, 19,
    39, 41, 56, 88, 99, 111, 116,
    169–188, 232
equine-assisted therapy, *xxxi*,
    42, 120
executive functioning, *xxiv, xxvii*,
    92, 172, 180, 184, 237, 274
expressive language, 90, 110, 113,
    183, 208, 234, 243, 264
eye contact, *xx*, 2, 6, 8, 12, 28–29,
    34, 55, 92, 103, 108, 115, 139,
    211, 217, 265

failure to thrive, *xx*, 41, 110, 274
feeding therapy, *xxx*, 49, 55, 113, 160
Finch, David, 90
First Steps, 3, 4, 8, 11, 44, 45, 50, 57–58, 106, 109, 125, 195
Fitzgerald, F. Scott, 259
floortime, 53, 274
food jags, *xxvii*, 274
Free and Appropriate Public Education (FAPE), 177
friendships, *xxi*, 118–119, 198, 224, 235, 245–246, 264
gastroenterologist, *xxx*, 39, 57
gastrointestinal system, 9, 30, 31
genetic counseling, 45, 64, 67

Ginott, Haim, 174
Grandin, Temple (PhD), 36, 39, 90, 96, 124, 174, 226, 228, 283–286
Greene, Vivian, 146
gross motor skills, 4, 6, 121
guardian ad litem (GAL), 162, 191
Gymboree Play and Music, 25, 31

Hague, Jason, 95
haircuts, 37
Hall, Elaine, 203
Halladay, Alycia (PhD), 13
Hampton, Kelle, 93
Hartley, Sigan (PhD), 149
hidden curriculum, 232, 243, 266, 274
High Ability Program, *xxiii*, *xxvi*, 119, 225
high-functioning autism, *xi*, *xxii*, 92, 99, 224, 273
holidays, 129–138
Hoopmann, Kathy, 283
"Human" (Perri), 248
hygiene, 238

hyperlexia, 116, 274

identity first, *xi*
imaginative play, 29, 55
In a Different Key: The Story of Autism (Donvan and Zucker), 93, 284
inclusion, 177–178, 275
Indiana Resource Center for Autism (IRCA), 89, 255
Individualized Education Plan (IEP), *xxiii*, 14, 106, 109, 112, 117, 171, 173, 177–181, 187–188, 275
Individuals with Disabilities Education Act (IDEA), 176
interoception, 103, 275

joint attention, 28, 30, 33, 55, 275
Journal of Best Practices (Finch), 90

Kanner, Leo (MD), 96
Karp, Harvey (MD), 30
Ketchup is My Favorite Vegetable: A Family Grows Up With Autism (Carter), 67, 154, 284
Kingsley, Emma Pearl, 60
Knost, L. R., 101

learned helplessness, 238, 275
least restrictive environment (LRE), 177, 245
Life, Animated (Suskind), 92, 124, 258, 285
Light and Life, *xxxi*, 114–115
Lovaas, Ivar (PhD), 182
low-functioning autism, *xi*, *xx*

Magnetic Resonance Imaging (MRI), *xxx*, 57

Magro, Kerry, *xix*, 95, 256, 286
mainstreaming, 177, 275
Making Peace with Autism: One Family's Story of Struggle, Discovery, and Unexpected Gifts (Senator), 74–75, 90, 126, 254
Medicaid waiver programs, 74–75, 90, 126, 254
medication, 46, 123, 180, 186
meltdowns, 34, 36, 58, 72–73, 87–88, 92, 121–124, 130, 132, 136–137, 140, 143, 191, 200, 220, 225, 240
midline, 50, 133, 275
mind-blindness, 212, 233, 264, 275
mirror neurons, 232, 275
modifications, 22, 90, 114, 119, 172,175, 188
motor plan, 28, 47, 50–53, 55, 58, 71, 74, 113, 183, 238, 243, 275–276
muscle tone, 4

neurodiversity, *xi*
neurologist, *xxi, xxix-xxx*, 4–7, 9–11, 35, 45, 50, 57, 59, 67, 106, 109, 119, 154
Neurotribes (Silberman), 92
Notbohm, Ellen, 169, 182, 285

occupational therapy, *xxii, xxix*, 1, 3–4, 37, 46–50, 56, 61, 118, 133, 151, 170, 176, 195
The Oprah Winfrey Show, 153
oral sensory dysfunction, 39, 47–48, 239, 276
O'Toole, Jennifer, 90, 227, 233, 285–286

Parenthood, 79, 156, 217, 286
Parents, coping strategies, 59
Pausch, Randy, 43
Perri, Christina, 248
pediatrician, *xxix-xxx*, 2–5, 7, 9–10, 35, 44, 51, 57, 63, 106, 142, 176, 194–195
perseveration, 28, 125, 242, 276
pervasive developmental disorder (PDD), *xxix*, 3, 8, 194–195, 276
Pervasive Developmental Disorder-Not Otherwise Specified (PDD-NOS), 3, 276
physical therapy, *xxix*, 3, 4, 44, 50–53, 176
Picture Exchange Communication System (PECS), 53, 110, 114–115,262, 276
plasticity of brain, *xxii*
Play-N-Share, *xxxi*, 112–113, 115–116
post-traumatic stress disorder (PTSD), 155
Pratt, Cathy (PhD), 89
Prizant, Barry (PhD), 92, 113, 152, 229, 236, 285–286
procedural safeguards, 109, 170, 177
proprioception, 28, 47–48, 51, 55, 101, 238, 276

Rain Man, 123, 183, 285
receptive language, 90, 110, 113–114, 207, 234, 243, 264
refrigerator mothers, 96
regression, 9, 29–30, 33, 112
retreat room, 132, 134
Rett syndrome, 3–4, 8–9, 11, 277

Riley Children's Hospital, 8, 12, 49, 52, 80, 99, 140, 167, 260

Robison, John Elder, 178, 230–231, 235, 285–286, 292

Rothschild, Chloe, 90

Sally-Anne Test, 233

self-advocacy, 188, 241, 266

self-regulation, 3, 176, 265, 277

Senator, Susan, 92, 95, 285–286

sensory diet, 47, 277

sensory modulation, 1, 46–47, 132, 277

sensory processing disorder, *xxii*, 4, 6, 11, 47, 110, 131, 133, 143, 276–277

Shakespeare, William, 239

Shore, Stephen (ED), 93, 241, 244, 265, 285–286

siblings, *xxviii*, 63–81, 145, 202, 255

Sibshops, 75

Silberman, Steve, 92

single motherhood, 149–168

Sisterhood of the Spectrum: An Asperger Chick's Guide to Life (O'Toole), 90, 227, 285

social/play therapy, *xxxi*, 56

social pragmatics, *xviii*, *xxvii*, 41, 172, 180, 183, 213, 225, 264, 277

Social Stories, 49, 277

Somatization Disorder, 110, 277

special education law, 88, 172, 176

special needs ministry, 97

speech therapy, *xxx*, 3, 53, 61, 118, 176

splinter skills, 243, 277

starfall.com, 115, 151

stimming, *xx*, 3, 120, 172, 264–265, 277

support groups, 59, 75, 87–89, 98, 156, 174, 196–197

Suresteps, *xxx*, 51

Suskind, Cornelia, 258

Suskind, Owen, 124

Suskind, Ron, 92, 124, 127

swallow/feeding study, *xxx*, 39, 57, 68, 259

Teacher of Record (TOR), 117, 175, 188, 267

teeth brushing, 11, 33, 68, 176, 238–239

Ten Things Your Student With Autism Wishes You Knew (Notbohm), 182, 285

text boxes, 6, 22, 29, 42, 46, 55, 59, 70, 78, 95, 104–105, 132, 141, 160, 167, 180, 186, 200, 217–218, 225, 236, 245, 263–266

The Asperkid's Secret Book of Social Rules (O'Toole), 227, 285

The Big Bang Theory, 149, 286

The Happiest Baby on the Block (Karp), 30

theory of mind, *xxiv*, 233, 275, 277

The Way I See It (Grandin), 174, 284

toilet training, 50, 105, 176, 186, 250

Tolleson, Michael, 12, 58, 92, 184, 186, 240

triggers, 93

twice-exceptional (2e), 19, 225, 277

Uniquely Human (Prizant), 93, 113, 152, 229, 285

upper body strength, 26, 28, 32, 50, 117, 120, 122

vacations, 23, 59, 129, 131,
    138–147, 157–158, 229, 267
Vaughn, Sarah, 243
verbal sequences, 238
vestibular sense, 47, 51, 265, 278
video modeling, 48, 110, 278

Warner, Jason (PhD), 160
Welcome to Holland (Kingsley), 60
Wheeler, Marci, 255
Wilbarger Brushing Protocol, 247

window of time, *xxii*, 41
Winner, Michelle Garcia, 90
Wisdom from the Round Table,
    xxiv-xxviii, 14, 23, 37, 61, 80,
    98, 127, 147, 167, 187, 200,
    218, 250, 266
Wooten, Linda, 15
working memory, 237, 278

Zoom (Cummings, S.), 90
Zucker, Karen, 93, 284

acknowledgments

First and foremost, thank you to Hannah and Connor. I will forever be grateful to both of you for allowing me to share our intimate story. The ink is not yet dry. The *Taylor Trio* has more chapters to write. Let's see how exciting we can make them!

The most influential individual in bringing our family's story to the page has been my book coach and friend, Ann Kroeker. Her incomparable acumen for the writing process is beyond words. Ann's passion for my endeavor to write the book that I could never find encouraged me beyond words. Her dynamic personality and love of the written word was a tremendous asset. She always had Hannah and the reader in mind. I thank her dearly for guiding me to find my voice and angle to inspire others to spread awareness and advocacy. I am blessed our paths crossed. *Dragonfly* would not exist in the form it is today without Ann.

My sincere appreciation and respect to the ladies who comprised the Wisdom from the Round Table. I'll never forget our first evening together and the truths that were shared. Your experiences allowed *Dragonfly* to reach a wider audience and encourage a larger scope of readers. I was in good company.

I appreciate the entire team at Skyhorse Publishing for believing in me and dedicating titles related to autism. I thank Tony Lyons (fellow parent with a daughter on the spectrum), Skyhorse Publishing's President and Publisher, for reading *Dragonfly's* proposal and taking a leap of faith, Louise Conte for acquiring the title, and Jody Faulkner for our time together in New Orleans. A special word of gratitude to my editor, Michael Campbell, for his clear vision, editorial style, and the ability to polish my prose with tender loving care.

Autism awareness and advocacy have come a long way in the last few decades due to the tireless commitment of others who ensured that our children wouldn't be marginalized. I thank Bernard Rimland, Ruth Sullivan, Lorna Wing, Temple Grandin, Jennifer O'Toole, John Elder Robison, and many others.

Chapter 14, *A New Day*, wouldn't have been on my family's horizon if it weren't for my exceptional warriors—too many to list. I will never forget what each of you did for my family.

My parents, James and Brenda Ashley, have given us their unwavering love and support. They have always acknowledged my potential and successes and helped me survive my ups and downs. Thanks to my mom for the late-night read-throughs.

Lilly Endowment helped to bring my dream to fruition by awarding me with a Teacher Creativity Fellowship Grant. Without this funding, I may have never had a literary archive for my children and a resource for parents with children on the spectrum.

Last of all is a thanks to my students that have graced the chairs in my classroom throughout my journey. Thanks for listening to all of my stories, respecting my most important story, understanding, and all the dragonfly mementoes.

about the author

Lori Ashley Taylor is a nationally recognized speaker on autism, founder of local autism support groups, founder and publisher of the website *Emerging from Autism*, and a tireless advocate offering insight and encouragement to families struggling to know the next steps to take. She lives outside Indianapolis, Indiana, with her two children, Hannah and Connor. She is a public school teacher and enjoys her faith, exercise, travel, and soaking up her children's younger years.

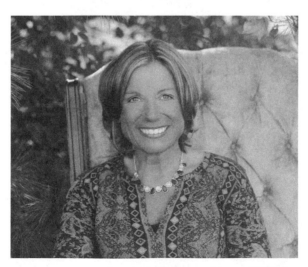

© 2016 by Loree Alayne Wheeler